Constructions of Disabilit

This innovative book discusses the meaning of 'inclusion' through the exploration of the interactions between disabled and non-disabled people at a community leisure centre. By exploring the nature of this interface an understanding of how people create the potential for both disability and inclusion is revealed. Thus this book takes a very different approach to that of existing texts, which have tended to concentrate mainly on disabled people's exclusion. The advantage of this new approach is that it adds an extra dimension to our understanding of how discriminatory practice is variously perpetuated and challenged. This book does not seek to undermine existing disability study texts, but rather to extend the focus of disability research to the ways that activity in the disabled and non-disabled interface is implicated in reinforcing or challenging oppression.

The book is valuable reading for all people who are working towards increased social inclusion for disabled people, including theorists and students of disability studies and learning difficulty, leisure management and disability service providers, and disabled people and their families. Using a practical case study approach, it explores the impact that social interaction between disabled and non-disabled people can have in increasing or decreasing disabled people's opportunities for inclusion. Examples of both inclusive and discriminatory practice are described in detail, and their positive and negative effects are demonstrated and discussed. This book offers a wide range of practical suggestions for the future development of more inclusive theory, policy and practice.

Claire Tregaskis is a researcher with the Inclusive Education and Equality Research Centre at the University of Sheffield. Her research is influenced by her previous experience as a countryside disability access adviser, and utilizes a combination of theoretical, practitioner and user perspectives in seeking new ways of generating the potential for greater social inclusion for disabled people.

Constructions of Disability

Researching the interface between
disabled and non-disabled people

Claire Tregaskis

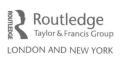

Routledge
Taylor & Francis Group

LONDON AND NEW YORK

E·S·R·C
ECONOMIC
& SOCIAL
RESEARCH
COUNCIL

First published 2004
by Routledge
II New Fetter Lane, London EC40 4EE

Simultaneously published in the USA and Canada
by Routledge
29 West 35th Street, New York, NY 10001

Routledge is an imprint of the Taylor & Francis Group

Typeset in Sabon and Gill by BC Typesetting Ltd, Bristol
Printed and bound in Great Britain by
MPG Books Ltd, Bodmin

British Library Cataloguing in Publication Data
A catalogue record for this book is available from the British Library

Library of Congress Cataloging in Publication Data
A catalog record has been requested

ISBN 0–415–32182–4 (hbk)
ISBN 0–415–32183–2 (pbk)

To my Aged Ps, who made everything in my life possible

Contents

14 Conclusions   138

Acknowledgements

First and foremost, deepest thanks are due to the staff and customers of Greenways Leisure Centre, without whose participation the research on which this book is based would not have been possible. Equally important was the ongoing advice and support provided by my research supervisor, Peter Clough, and that of the other members of my research support group – Mairtin Mac an Ghaill, Pippa Murray, Cathy Nutbrown and Uri Rennie. Without their ongoing encouragement and practical advice I know there were times when I might easily have given up on the project, and taken up something less challenging instead, like white water rafting or marathon running. Also, in a very practical sense, I couldn't have completed this work without my support workers, to whom my thanks are also due. So, now that I've finally got to the end of it, this book is for all of you.

In addition, the support of the Economic and Social Research Council (Awards R00429834720 and T026271110) in funding both the research phase of this project and the subsequent writing-up is gratefully acknowledged; as are the journals *Disability and Society* and *Managing Leisure*, for granting permission for me to reproduce some material here that has previously appeared in their publications. For further information on this, readers are referred to the Taylor & Francis website, www.tandf.co.uk.

Chapter 1

Introduction

What this book is about

This book explores some of the ways in which constructions of disability can affect disabled people's chances of inclusion in ordinary mainstream social environments. Through a detailed investigation of social interactions between disabled and non-disabled people in one such setting – a leisure centre – it explores a range of factors that can affect people's ability to relate to each other, and what parts both individual and structural constructions of disability can play in the ongoing process of creating inclusion and exclusion. In so doing, the book demonstrates some of the ways in which people may use disability and impairment as reasons to either put up barriers between themselves and others, or as the basis of establishing common ground, depending on the situation and the circumstances in which they find themselves.

At the outset I should explain that, although the research discussed here took place in a recreational setting, and the data was collected using a range of ethnographic research methods, this book is not a conventional ethnographic study of a leisure centre. In other words, it will not tell you everything you ever wanted to know about how a leisure centre operates, nor does it offer a detailed analysis of the economics and politics of leisure provision in Britain today, although these issues are touched upon in some of the discussion that follows. Instead, the leisure centre here forms a situational backdrop to the relationships between disabled and non-disabled people which are the primary focus of this research. In this account, it is principally those interactions that are foregrounded and analysed, and not the setting as a whole. This is achieved largely through the relatively unusual device of using myself as simultaneously researcher and research subject, and by recording the ways in which disability was constructed through other people's responses to me and to the other disabled people I met in the course of the research. As a result, what follows is in part an exploration of who I was in that setting. By deconstructing my multiple identities at the leisure centre, I will show something of the complexity of who I was in that setting, as well as uncovering some of the ways that non-disabled people's multiple identities were equally implicated in the range of ways in which they responded to me and to the other disabled people they encountered. The study thus aims to disrupt the apparent certainties of one-dimensional cause-and-effect analyses of disabled people's exclusion by showing that, in this setting at least, the jumble of interpersonal relationships combined with the impact of the politics and economics of the leisure centre made for a far more complex and confusing scenario. The findings suggest that there are no 'quick fixes' in terms of challenging exclusion, but that instead a range of situationally appropriate access solutions is required before real inclusion may be said to have been achieved.

Refocusing on the interface between disabled and non-disabled people

In focusing explicitly on the dynamics of the interpersonal interface between disabled and non-disabled people as a means of exploring the possibilities for inclusion, this work differs from previous disability-related texts that have concentrated primarily on reporting disabled people's response to the experience of oppression. That wider task of demonstrating disabled people's exclusion from mainstream structures such as education, housing, the world of work, and other areas of social interaction which members of the mainstream take for granted has already been ably undertaken by others (e.g. Barnes, 1991; Barton, 1993; Clough and Barton, 1998; Mason and Rieser, 1999; Oliver, 1990, 1996; Simons, 1992; Vernon, 1999), and this study does not seek to replicate their findings as such. Instead, by exploring the disabled/non-disabled interface in more detail, the research aims to expose the subtlety of some forms of disability discrimination from a different angle, including an analysis of the part which both disabled and non-disabled people may play in variously replicating and challenging exclusionary policies, practices and behaviours (Giroux, 1992).

This focus on the interface follows a recent wider trend of researching previously taken-for-granted categories as a means of challenging oppression. Thus Stanley and Wise (1993: 31) argue that 'any analysis of women's oppression *must* involve research on the part played by men in this'. In similar vein, Kitzinger and Wilkinson (1993) have questioned the assumption that heterosexuality is the norm in feminist theory, and contributors to their collection have sought to problematize their own heterosexuality. Equally, Wong (1994) has exposed whiteness as an uncontested category in research, and Tarver-Behring (1994: 207) has called upon white women to acknowledge and explore the multiplicity of their own identities as a precursor to being able to better understand – and make connections with – women from minority groups, who of course have equally complex and multiple identities. This book follows this new trend of minorities investigating majorities as a way of adding to our understanding of the reasons for the ongoing prevalence of discrimination against minority groups in Western societies. Many instances of discrimination are documented and presented for analysis here. However, the data also suggest that there may be some cause for cautious optimism, by questioning traditional assumptions of a binary and unchangeable opposition between all aspects of disabled and non-disabled people's experiences, and thereby allowing for the possibility of identifying limited common ground on which to base practical alliances for change.

Indeed, one of the purposes of this book is to encourage disabled and non-disabled people to explore some of the ways in which their own actions may (often unconsciously) compound the exclusion of others. In writing it, I have been forced to challenge my own prior assumption that non-disabled people have the monopoly on oppressive behaviour. Instead, as the data discussed here will show, we all have the capacity to oppress people who are situationally less powerful than us (Vernon, 1999). However, it remains the case that, although sometimes protected from particular instances of oppression by their class, gender, race, ethnicity and sexual orientation (Appleby, 1993, 1994; Corbett, 1994; Humphrey, 2000; Vernon, 1999), disabled people are in general one of the most oppressed groups in British society (Barnes, 1991). Thus there are detailed here many instances of interactions characterized by the operation of unequal power relations, in which the person with less situational power was usually also a disabled person. However, also discussed are examples of disabled and non-disabled people coming together on an equal basis to achieve a common goal, a cooperative model of working that may point the way towards a common future based on mutual respect and the equal valuing of difference.

Why I wanted to write this book

My research focus here on exploring some of the practicalities involved in working towards achieving greater social inclusion came about largely as a result of events in my own life as a disabled person. Although I attended mainstream schools throughout my education, it was by no means a happy experience, and by the time I left school I was convinced that non-disabled people were a different species of being to me, and that we had nothing in common with each other. However, once my working life began, I found that the vast majority of people with whom I was working were members of this non-disabled alien species. Since I could not avoid contact altogether, I realized that I had to find common ground with at least some of them if my time at work was not to be incredibly lonely and isolated. And then over the years, as both my self-confidence and my professional work skills increased, so too I realized that my personal relationships with non-disabled people had actually become an important, even necessary, part of my existence. They were no longer aliens – now they were my friends – and in many respects our commonality had become as important as our differences.

Undertaking the research on which this book is based gave me the opportunity to reflect back on those formative years and, in seeking to uncover something of non-disabled people's approach to disability issues, also forced me to review my communication strategies, and the ways in which my own behaviour has variously challenged or perpetuated existing prejudice against both disabled and non-disabled people. As such it was not an entirely comfortable process, but it did teach me a great deal about myself. In undertaking this journey, and in uncovering examples of prejudice against more than just disabled people, I also found myself moving from a fairly solid disability studies mindset to one which sits somewhere in the interface of explanations for a range of oppressions including disablism, sexism and racism. Therefore, although the ostensible focus of this book lies in exploring constructions of disability, both its research approach and its findings make it relevant not just to a traditional disability studies audience, but also to the wider readership of policy makers and practitioners who are similarly engaged in the process of trying to develop inclusive practice.

Aims of the book

In the context of developing social policy aimed at achieving inclusion for all minority groups, the book has four main objectives.

- First, it will show that bringing about more inclusive practice is about changing attitudes as well as adapting organizational policies and practices.
- Second, in focusing on the disabled/non-disabled interface it will show what non-disabled people in one social setting – anonymized here as 'Greenways Leisure Centre' to protect its real identity – thought about disability, impairment and disabled people, as well as something of what they thought about women and people from minority ethnic groups.
- Third, it will question the implicit assumption in many existing social model of disability accounts of a permanent and unchanging binary opposition between the interests and experiences of disabled and non-disabled people, and will suggest that actually we may have more in common than we think.
- Fourth, the complex and often contradictory nature of the findings reported here disrupts the apparent certainties of one-dimensional cause-and-effect analyses of inclusion and exclusion, and suggests instead that a range of situationally appropriate access solutions is required before real inclusion may be said to have been achieved.

Why focus on leisure in this research?

Choosing to base research into disabled/non-disabled interactions at a leisure centre might at first sight appear an odd decision, when social settings such as schools and workplaces are more usually in the forefront of discussions about how inclusion for disabled people can be achieved. However, there were a number of reasons for my choice of location. First, because disabled people are at least three times as likely as non-disabled people to be unemployed (Vernon, 1999) it seemed unrealistic to locate the research in a workplace setting where there might be few or no disabled members of staff, and/or where there was little or no contact with members of the public. Similarly, I expected that there would be relatively few disabled children and staff in mainstream schools. At a leisure centre, however, it was assumed that there would be enough disabled people present to make it possible to observe a sufficient amount and variety of social interactions between them and non-disabled people to enable research conclusions to be drawn from the data.

Second, the recent explosive growth of the leisure industry, especially in areas of the country where traditional heavy industry has declined, combined with demographic changes resulting in a higher proportion of older people in the population as a whole, means that the need to ensure that leisure provision takes account of the needs of older and/or disabled people is increasingly relevant to policy makers and practitioners alike (Torkildsen, 1993: 1.19). Further, new research into young disabled people's experiences of leisure provision (Murray, 2002) undertaken in parallel with the present study, shows that they see leisure as being central to their individual experiences of inclusion and exclusion. Indeed, it is in such relatively less formal leisure settings that the presence or absence of the sort of social networks and relationships that most members of the mainstream can take for granted may either create new opportunities for disabled young people's enjoyment and personal growth, or else starkly reinforce their feelings of social isolation. This finding endorses recent legislative and policy developments relating to disabled people. Both the 1995 Disability Discrimination Act and the 2001 White Paper *Valuing People: A New Strategy for Learning Disability for the 21st Century* require policy makers and service providers concerned with developing and delivering services of all kinds to respond creatively to the access needs of disabled people, who form an important and sizeable customer market. Of particular relevance to this study are the provisions made in Part III of the Disability Discrimination Act, which place a legal duty on those providing goods, facilities and services to the public to avoid discriminating against disabled people. Thus, since December 1996 it has been unlawful for service providers to treat disabled people less favourably than non-disabled people on the basis of impairment. Since October 1999, service providers have had a duty to make what are termed 'reasonable adjustments' to their service delivery, if disabled people need this in order to be able to access the service; and, from 2004, reasonable adjustments will also have to be made to improve physical access to venues. Also pertinent here is the need referred to in the *Valuing People* White Paper (Department of Health, 2001: 80) for disability service providers to include access to leisure activities as an integral part of individual and community care plans, rather than viewing this as a non-essential optional extra, as is often the case at present.

Finally, at a personal level my decision to base the research in a leisure setting resulted directly from my previous professional background as a countryside recreation officer, where my job had involved bringing together recreation managers and disabled people to plan and implement the removal of physical and programme access barriers. For this research project I knew that I wanted to study relationships in an area of the leisure industry, but not within the countryside setting with which I was perhaps too familiar. I hoped that choosing a leisure centre for the research instead would enable me to bring to this new setting some of my pre-existing generic recreation manage-ment skills and knowledge, whilst also providing me with the opportunity to observe additional management techniques that were new to me. I was also interested to explore whether an indoor leisure setting would prove as relaxed and inclusive as I had found many countryside management services to be.

In presenting my research data on interactions between disabled and non-disabled people at Greenways Leisure Centre, I hope to reinforce Murray's (2002) finding that participation in leisure is of central importance to disabled people's experiences of inclusion and exclusion, because of the interplay involved between the desire for access to leisure and the need for inclusive social relationships to help put this desire into practice. This is the essential extra human dimension that we sometimes miss when we concentrate solely on reacting to legislative and policy imperatives without understanding exactly why such developments are important in the lives of real people. I hope that the research findings presented here will help to underscore why disabled people need better access to leisure, as well as suggesting some practical ways in which this can be achieved.

Constructions of disability: the link between structural and attitude barriers

Carrying out research within a leisure setting used by disabled and non-disabled people alike proved to be a useful fulcrum point for studying diver-sity, discrimination and cooperation in action. Through an investigation of the construction of disability within that setting, I was able to explore the hypothesis that such responses, and the attitudes that flow from them, do not exist in isolation but are in fact created, altered and maintained by a wide range of external material and cultural factors, as well as by individual psychological ones. I wanted to see if it was possible to resituate the 'attitude problem' from the realm of the purely personal to where I believe it truly belongs – simultaneously in the interface between individual disabled and non-disabled people, and in the positioning of those individual relationships within a wider historically specific social context of political, economic and administrative inclusionary–exclusionary influences (see also Thomas (1999)). I believe that making such a shift in emphasis would in turn make it more difficult for discrimination's apologists to continue to explain exclusionary practice on the grounds of impairment as resulting purely from an individual's failure to understand 'the other' because of their perceived difference from the non-disabled norm. In pursing an agenda for disabled people's inclusion, then, this book will make the case that attitude-based discrimination should be viewed as forming an equal part of a symbiotic, mutually sustaining, relationship with structural-based discrimination. Later chapters will show some of the ways in which attitudinal and structural barriers were uncovered and challenged in the research setting. In turn, these data form the basis of my main argument here, which is that attitudinal and structural barriers must be addressed simultaneously in order to make sustained and timely progress, rather than assuming that either structural change or attitudinal change alone will end discrimination against disabled people. Thus we need to get to a position where disability discrimination is viewed as being on a par with other forms of social oppression, including institutionalized racism (Home Office, 1999), and begins to be tackled in a similarly systematic way across all social structures.

Organization of the remainder of this book

It is recognized that the readership for this book is drawn from a range of professional and practitioner fields. Thus the main body of the text starts in Chapter 2 with an introduction to those ideas from the disability field, specifically the social model of disability and normalization/Social Role Valorization, that have influenced both the way in which the research was carried out, and the subsequent data analysis. Chapter 3 continues the focus on theory, by examining how and why my analysis of the construction of disability was made easier once I had recognized the importance of multiple identity as a key medium through which disabled people's exclusion at Greenways was variously perpetuated and challenged. Moving more toward the practical, also discussed here is my growing awareness of the ways in which my own presence in, and influence on, events at the leisure centre affected the research; and the way that over time I came to view the inevitability of this 'researcher effect' on the field of study as adding an extra dimension to my understanding of the way in which disability is variously constructed and challenged through the attribution and/or projection of particular aspects of an individual's identity in social settings.

It was this discovery of the vital importance of identity formation and attribution in improving or diminishing the potential for inclusion that led to the identity-related structuring of subsequent chapters of the book. Thus Chapters 4 to 13 chart my observation and understanding of a range of inclusive and exclusionary practices as revealed to me through the complexity of my own multiple identities as researcher, consultant, member of staff, friend, woman, white person, embodied being, disabled person, oppressor and activist. In each of these chapters I have selected and described key events which seemed to illustrate people's constructions of disability in that situation, depending on their perceptions of my identity at the time. In some chapters there is relatively little directly attributable data, while others have a lot. I have decided, however, to keep them all in, so as to reflect as fully as possible the complexity of my fieldwork identities and relationships. Sometimes indeed it proved impossible to completely separate out one identity from another, and in those situations an element of cross-referencing and replication of data has proved inevitable. In all these chapters, I show what people's existing attitudes were, and then go on to give some suggestions as to ways in which policy and practice might be developed in the future so as to reduce the occurrence of disability and increase the potential for inclusion. Finally, a brief explanation of the ordering of these data chapters is required. Given that not all readers will have personal experience of impairment, or of impairment-related disability, I decided to start with chapters which discussed those aspects of my identity which were in themselves the least overtly impairment-related. It is hoped that both disabled and non-disabled readers will discover some aspects of my experiences here, for example around being a researcher, a friend, or a woman, with which they can consciously identify. As the book progresses, I then move on to discuss issues around the impaired body, and being both a disabled person and an oppressor, which may be less familiar to some readers. I end the data analysis on what is deliberately intended to be a positive note, by describing my experiences of activism in challenging exclusion and bringing about change within the setting, before moving on in the final chapter to a discussion of my general conclusions and some of the possible implications for the future development of theory, policy and practice around inclusion that have arisen from this research.

Chapter 2

Researching the interface

Theories on the construction of disability

Analytical framework: an introduction to the social model of disability

In trying to understand and analyse interactions between disabled and non-disabled people at Greenways I took as my starting point the analytical framework provided by the social model of disability. Since their initial development in the 1970s, social model ideas have become a crucially important explanatory tool for those disabled people who have developed and been touched by the disabled people's movement, not least for me in my own life and in conducting the research for this book. Social model explanations of disability represent a different way of explaining disabled people's oppression from previous medicalized accounts, because for the first time they have suggested that many of the problems disabled people face are caused not by their impairments, but rather because society is organized in a way that does not take their needs into account. In turn, this holistic vision of disabled people's oppression implies that, if society is implicated in perpetuating this state of affairs, so all members of that society also have the potential to challenge exclusion, both in our positioning as individuals – by learning to act more inclusively around each other – and in our professional roles as legislators, policy makers and practitioners, in which we may have the power to introduce changes that increase the potential for inclusion. Thus challenging disabled people's exclusion changes from being a cause of concern solely for individual disabled people and their families and advocates, and instead becomes a social duty in which all members of society are implicated. On this interpretation, the social model approach is a profoundly optimistic one, because it recognizes that to achieve change requires that we expect the best of people in acting in ways that challenge existing oppressive practice.

This belief is not based on naivety on my part, but rather on fifteen years' previous experience as a countryside access officer, in which I routinely worked with countryside managers and disabled people to implement social model solutions to a range of physical and programme access problems. In that specific service setting, the potential for social model approaches to increase the more general potential for wider social inclusion was revealed, in that access solutions designed primarily with disabled people's needs in mind also improved provision for all other visitors (BT/ The Fieldfare Trust, 1997). Thus the application of social model ideas to practitioner settings has potential benefits for everyone, not just disabled people. Accordingly, in terms of this new research it provided the most appropriate framework within which to discuss the interface between disabled and non-disabled people, the varied and conflicting roles they may play in variously perpetuating and challenging oppression, and whether and how bringing about truly inclusive policies and practices is achievable in service settings.

The difference between 'disability' and 'impairment'

Since social model ideas pervade the explanations for discrimination against disabled people given in this book, before going further it may be helpful to review the main strands of social model thinking. Central to the social model is the belief that, in contemporary Britain, people with impairments are disabled/excluded by a society which is not organized in a way which takes account of their needs (Finkelstein, 1980; Oliver, 1990, 1996; UPIAS, 1976). In social model thinking, then, a key distinction is drawn between the terms 'impairment' and 'disability', an analysis which represents a new way of thinking about the structure of oppression against disabled people. This distinction has been explained in the following terms by Disabled People's International, with wording subsequently adapted by Barnes for use in the United Kingdom context:

> *Impairment* is the functional limitation within the individual caused by physical, mental or sensory impairment. *Disability* is the loss or limitation of opportunities to take part in the normal life of the community on an equal level with others due to physical and social barriers.
>
> (1991: 2)

Here, a distinction is drawn between the acknowledged inherent functional limitations caused to the individual by their impairment, and the additional socially created barriers caused by disability. This distinction is based on a pragmatic recognition that people may face limitations in what they can do as a result of their impairments, while at the same time challenging the imposition of additional social barriers created by a society which does not take the needs of people with impairments into account, thereby further limiting their opportunities for full participation within that society.

Social model thinking thus requires that we analyse the problem of disabled people's social exclusion in new ways that avoid a victim-blaming approach. To give one practical example, before social model ideas were developed, if a wheelchair user could not get into a building, the building's owner could say 'What a shame you can't get into this building because you can't walk up the steps'. And most of the time disabled people would agree with this statement, because back then the main frame of reference available to explain their experience was the individual/medical model, which focuses on the functional limitations caused by people's individual impairments as being the main reason for their social exclusion. So everyone – both disabled and non-disabled people – bought into the idea that disabled people couldn't go to places or participate in activities because of 'what was wrong with them'. The trouble with this explanation was that it was really pessimistic. It seemed to offer disabled people no hope of greater social inclusion unless they could change themselves by getting rid of their impairments. But of course this isn't a practical option. The big difference that social model ideas have made is that they restate the problem in a different way. So, instead of saying, 'What a shame you can't get into this building because you can't walk up the steps', a social model approach would say 'Actually, you can't get into this building because it has been poorly designed'. The social model view, then, is that disability is caused by human factors, like a building being poorly designed, or an organizational promotions policy that puts disabled employees at a disadvantage compared to their non-disabled colleagues. Thus disability is not a characteristic of, or the fault of, individual people with impairments, but is instead a term used to describe all the extra difficulties that people with impairments face because society is not organized in ways that take their needs into account. As such, the social model definition of disability is potentially a more positive tool for change than the individual medical model approach, because it suggests that disability could be eradicated if society was organized in ways that took the needs of all its citizens into account. In relation to this book, then, when I talk about 'constructions of disability', my focus is on the additional social barriers that people with impairments face, and how these exclusionary mechanisms might be overcome.

Main strands of social model thinking

Supporting this central belief that people with impairments experience additional oppression because of the exclusionary way that society is currently organized, is a range of additional explanations that illustrate and expand upon the baseline thesis. To date, the most influential social model explanation has been the modernist materialist one, which argues that people with impairments have come to face a specific and explicit form of exclusion under modern capitalism, and suggests that social inclusion will be achieved once the exclusionary capitalist system is replaced by a more equitable social system (Finkelstein, 1980; Oliver, 1990, 1996; Thomas, 1999). In recent years other explanations have also been put forward. Both materialists and post-structuralists have explored and highlighted the importance of the culture and media of the society in justifying and maintaining the exclusion of those defined as 'other' (Abberley, 1987, 1997; Barnes, 1991, 1996; Hevey, 1992; Shakespeare, 1994). Others have argued that some forms of impairment, including mild and moderate learning difficulty, in fact have no organic origin, and have instead been wholly culturally created for political reasons, often as a means of labelling as 'other' people whose opportunities for educational progression have been limited by their class position. Giving them a socially devalued label in this way is thus intended to reduce the threat they are perceived to pose to mainstream society (Borthwick, 1996; Gelb, 1987; Manion and Bersani, 1987).

Feminist readings of disabled people's exclusion have questioned those social model analyses that appear to deliberately avoid any discussion of disabled people's subjective experience, or the integration of lessons drawn from that experience into social model theory (Marks, 1999a, 1999b; Morris, 1991, 1996; Thomas, 1999). Further, Walmsley (2001) has warned that a theory-level rejection of personal experience narratives may particularly exclude people with learning difficulties, whose experience of disablist oppression is currently often expressed primarily through the mediums of biography and life history, from contributing to the future development of social model ideas. There have also been calls to integrate an analysis of the impaired body at theory level (Crow, 1996; Hughes and Paterson, 1997; Paterson and Hughes, 1999), partly in recognition of parallel developments within mainstream sociology of theories about the body (for example, Glassner, 1992; Shilling, 1993; Turner, 1992), and also in response to an apparent concern that disability theory is in danger of becoming too inward-looking and self-referential (Barnes, Mercer and Shakespeare, 1999).

In discussing social model ideas, it is worth adding the rider that one of the 'fathers' of the social model, Mike Oliver, never claimed that the social model was designed to give a neat holistic explanation for all aspects of disabled people's exclusion, but was instead intended as a starting point for discussion of the issues. Despite his reservations, however, it might be argued that in practice the social model has in a sense come to act as a straitjacket for disabled people's experience (Oliver, 1996: 31). More positively, there is a strong case to be made in support of the contention that later additions to the original economics-based social model have extended its explanatory power, and increased its relevance to a wider range of disabled people. Such additions include analyses of the exclusionary power of contemporary culture (Aspis, 1999; Barnes, 1996; Hevey, 1992; Priestley, 1998; Shakespeare, 1994), attempts to develop a sociology of impairment (Hughes and Paterson, 1997; Paterson and Hughes, 1999), and a call for the recognition of the real psycho-emotional effects of disability (Thomas, 1999) in social model accounts. The need for disability theory to follow the example of the disability arts movement in actively celebrating the positive aspects of disabled people's experience has also recently been raised as an issue (Swain and French, 2000). Further ongoing theory-level developments are expected as social model writers continue to respond to changing expressions of oppression and discrimination against disabled people in Britain.

Although debate between people from different social model positions has often been fierce, in practical terms the social model has undoubtedly been an emancipatory concept in the lives of many disabled people (Campbell and Oliver, 1996; Germon, 1999; Thomas, 1999). Its ideas have given people the courage and self-belief to start to reclaim control of their lives through initiatives like the Independent Living Movement, taking direct action to bring their exclusion to the attention of the mainstream, and producing social model accounts of their history (Campbell and Oliver, 1996; Sutherland, 1981) which are both political and celebratory of their achievements – sometimes at the most basic level of refusing to 'conveniently' lie down and die. All this work is essential in making disabled people visible within society, and in moving towards a situation in which full civil rights and social inclusion are eventually achieved.

Normalization/Social Role Valorization accounts of the experience of people with learning difficulties

As has been demonstrated above, social model ideas differ from other explanations of disability in offering a social rather than an individual deficit approach to explaining the oppression that disabled people face. However, it is acknowledged that individual/medical model accounts remain influential in disability discourse. One area in which explanations for disabled people's experience is particularly contested is in the lives of people with learning difficulties, where theories of normalization/Social Role Valorization (SRV) have influenced the development of policy and practice for decades (Wolfensberger, 1992). In comparison to the normalization/SRV focus on the life experiences of people with learning difficulties, social model accounts have in the past been rightly criticized for failing to fully incorporate analysis of such experiences into their explanations for, and challenges to, disabled people's oppression (Chappell, 1998; Goodley and Moore, 2000; Chappell, Goodley and Lawthom, 2002).

In fact, a review of social model and normalization/SRV explanations of discrimination suggests significant similarity in their explanations of the ways in which society culturally discriminates against disabled people, and what effects this process may have on them (Barnes, 1996; Hevey, 1992; Oliver, 1990, 1996; Race, 1999; Shakespeare, 1994; Wolfensberger, 1992). However, these accounts then differ radically when it comes to developing approaches to achieving change aimed at improving disabled people's lives.

Thus, as previously discussed, the social model advocates a holistic structural barriers approach which focuses on bringing about changes to the
structure of society so that people with impairments are no longer viewed
as an unproductive drain on resources who face inevitable discrimination
as a result (Barnes, 1991; Finkelstein, 1980; Oliver, 1990, 1996; Thomas,
1999). Normalization/SRV as implemented in Britain and North America,
however, sees it as more realistic to concentrate on improving the lives of
disabled people (most commonly, people with learning difficulties) by encouraging their assimilation within the mainstream as a means of improving
their life chances; and views as well-meaning but unrealistic any attempt to
achieve wider social change (Race, 1999; Wolfensberger, 1992).

Of the two approaches, it is undoubtedly the case that normalization/SRV
has had the greater impact to date on the direction and development of
disability policies and practices. This is perhaps unsurprising, since it is an
approach developed and implemented by disability professionals who have
greater situational power, and hence more influence over policy and practice
in this field, than disabled people (Oliver, 1996). Thus normalization/SRV
principles have been key to legislative and policy developments relating to
disabled people over the past thirty years, including the 1971 DHSS Circular
Better Services for the Mentally Handicapped, the 1970 Education Act, the
1981 Green Paper and the 1983 Government Circular on Community Care,
the King's Fund programme *An Ordinary Life* (1980, 1984), and more
recently the 1995 Disability Discrimination Act and the 2001 White Paper
Valuing People. In the process, the ideological de-institutionalization focus
of normalization/SRV has been instrumental in encouraging policy makers
to enact the move from institutional to community care for many disabled
people (Brown and Smith, 1992). Normalization/SRV principles were also
influential in ensuring, through the 1970 Education Act, that for the first
time all disabled people had the right to an education (Tyne, 1992). Its
achievements are therefore of no small merit, and may rightly be said to
have changed the lives of many disabled people for the better.

However, just as some social model ideas have been criticized for a lack of
range, so the normalization/SRV approach to challenging disabled people's
social exclusion has been challenged from within the learning difficulty
field on several grounds. One area of debate has arisen around the normal-
ization/SRV 'conservative corollary' proposal (Wolfensberger, 1992). This
approach suggests that the most realistic way to challenge disabled people's
ongoing social exclusion is for disabled people to engage in a constant
process of self-regulation to avoid drawing attention to their perceived
difference and thereby increasing their chances of social acceptance, a
process previously described by Goffman (1990) as 'passing'. However,
this focus on encouraging individual disabled people to adapt to fit in with
existing social norms has been criticized for its basis in an historical deviancy

model, which assumes that disabled people will always be seen as unacceptably different from members of mainstream society, and will therefore always require the mediation of professional support to allow them to participate in society. Thus normalization/SRV has been described as a relatively static and conservative theory, in that it assumes things will always be as they are now, and does not critically evaluate or challenge the power relations inherent in professional–service user relationships which may actually make it difficult for disabled people to take control of their lives in the way that the normalization/SRV approach advocates. Critics have argued that in reality normative social values can and do change (Dalley, 1992; Whitehead, 1992). However, by perpetuating the devaluation of difference and encouraging conformity to existing normative values around appearance, behaviour and performance, normalization/SRV theory doesn't seem to allow for this possibility in relation to the way society sees disabled people.

Normalization/SRV has also been criticized for its recommendation that individuals with impairments should for preference mix with non-disabled people rather than with other 'devalued' disabled people, to minimize the negative feedback from members of the mainstream that may ensue from coming across a group of people who look different. This approach has been viewed as being unduly divisive, and lacking in recognition of the importance of developing a shared group identity and of belonging to a wider social movement of disabled people that celebrates difference rather than denying it (Szivos, 1992). Attention has also been drawn to the unconscious white male bias in normalization/SRV ideas, and the way in which issues of gender, class, sexuality and ethnicity have become obscured as a result (Brown and Smith, 1992; Walmsley and Downer, 1997; Williams and Nind, 1999).

Such criticism notwithstanding, the ongoing impact of normalization/SRV in the lives of people with learning difficulties remains influential. Indeed, its fierce critique of the shortcomings of much existing service provision for people with learning difficulties (Race, 1999; Wolfensberger, 1992) is a powerful indictment of service providers' ongoing failure to support disabled people's moves towards self-development and personal growth, expressed through the maintenance of organisational policies and practices that may actually reinforce disabled people's social exclusion instead of challenging it. In analysing instances of the exclusion of people with learning difficulties at Greenways, I will therefore draw on this aspect of normalization/SRV theory as an explanatory tool. However, the Greenways data also suggest limitations to the applicability of normalization/SRV approaches to challenging exclusion, because of its failure to recognize the extent to which the power of disability professionals is relatively uncontested in mainstream as well as in segregated settings. This research finding suggests that actually normalization/SRV strategies such as competency and image enhancement may be difficult to implement while disability professionals retain the power to keep disabled people separate from non-disabled people in mainstream settings. Overall, therefore, in analysing the research data I have found social model ideas more useful, because of their more holistic approach to charting and challenging disabled people's social exclusion.

Lessons for the social model from the experiences of people with learning difficulties

That said, it is undoubtedly true that social model thinkers have lessons to learn from the learning difficulty field. A major criticism of social model ideas from this quarter has been that little account has been taken in social model thinking of the ongoing influence of normalization/SRV on the lives of people with learning difficulties, and the knock-on effect this has had on their way of viewing themselves. As mentioned above, a key strategy adopted by normalization/SRV has been to attempt to promote the integration of people with learning difficulties into the mainstream by playing down their perceived difference from the non-disabled norm through the adoption of socially valued roles (Wolfensberger, 1992). Whether or not such an approach has in practice been successful – and there appears to be only limited empirical evidence of inclusion being achieved through this strategy alone (Szivos, 1992) – it has had a number of effects on the life experience and social expectations of people with learning difficulties. One such effect has been that many people with learning difficulties see the label of 'learning disability' as the specific cause of their oppression, rather than viewing this as simply another form of social barrier set up to divide people into more or less devalued groups. Another has been that some people with learning difficulties have internalized the normalization/SRV value that it is more socially acceptable, and more likely to lead to their own individual social integration, for them to mix with non-disabled people, than it is to associate with other disabled people (Dowse, 2001). Hence, as a result of their ongoing isolation from other disabled people, many people with learning difficulties have not yet recognized how labelling fits into the wider picture of oppression created by social barriers, or seen the value of developing solidarity with the wider disability movement (Walmsley, 1997).

Somewhat contentiously, it has also been argued that social model accounts focus too much on the experience of bodily impairment, which many people with learning difficulties do not see as relevant to their own lives (Chappell, Goodley and Lawthom, 2002; Walmsley, 2001). However, a different way of looking at this is offered by Gabel (1999) in discussing her own experience of living with mental illness, another form of impairment that is not always of the body. She argues that, for all of us, our bodies are always the medium through which we experience the world. Thus, even if our impairments are not of the body, everything we experience – including instances of oppression – comes to us when we are in our bodies, because we are all embodied beings. Hence it is less important to look at whether our impairments are of the body or of the mind, than it is to recognize our commonality of experience as embodied beings who are united by being on the receiving end of disablist oppression. In my view, this more holistic approach to viewing the impact of oppression on people's lives is one way in which deeper connections can be made between different disabled people's experiences.

These areas of ongoing debate highlight instances where specific links between the varying experiences of disability oppression have yet to be made. However, the need to develop such connections has been highlighted by Aspis (2002), who has highlighted the way in which the service provision focus of normalization/SRV has impacted on the development of the self-advocacy movement of people with learning difficulties. Her view is that self-advocacy has to a great extent been sidetracked into becoming a tool for measuring standards of existing service provision, rather than providing people with learning difficulties with a true means of empowerment by offering them the chance to 'think outside the box' and make different choices about what services they would like to see provided. In this way, she argues that the presence of ongoing structural barriers is obscured by the focus on tinkering with the details of existing provision. Small details of service provision may change as a result of such consultation, but the real power remains with the service providers to offer the services they think best. Aspis believes that actually true empowerment can only be achieved by people with learning difficulties forming alliances with the wider disability movement to tackle wider structural disabling barriers and oppressive power relations. In making such a statement, and arguing for a renewed focus by all disabled people on achieving wider structural change, it may be argued that the disabled people's movement is entering a more inclusive stage, in which a wider range of voices will be accorded equal value, and in which further theory-level developments more fully reflect the diverse interests and opinions of its constituency.

The application of social model ideas to this research

Throughout the rest of this book I will be making reference to social model ideas as I try to explain what I think was happening when disabled and non-disabled people came together at Greenways Leisure Centre. Where there was evidence of tangible structural barriers to inclusion (for example poor physical access, problems with information provision, and organizational policies which discriminated against disabled people) I will draw strongly on materialist social model accounts in suggesting ways in which those barriers might be overcome. However, in reviewing the literature I was disappointed to find very little discussion in social model writing about disabling attitudes and how to change them. For example, in his otherwise wide-ranging analysis of the shape and extent of institutionalized social, economic and political discrimination against disabled people in Britain, Barnes (1991) only devotes one page out of each 20–30 page chapter to discussing how non-disabled people's negative attitudes help to maintain disabled people's exclusion. Such an apparent underplaying of the disabling effects of negative attitudes persisted in much disability studies literature until as recently as 1999, when Thomas called for more discussion of the psycho-emotional effects of disabling attitudes within social model accounts.

To some extent I can understand why theorists have previously chosen to underplay the significance of negative attitudes as a cause of disabled people's exclusion. First, there is a real danger that attitudes come to be seen as the only barrier to inclusion, and that as a result nothing is then done to challenge more tangible (and financially more expensive) structural barriers. As the Greater Manchester Coalition of Disabled People put it in pointing out the failings of individualizing attitudes-focused approaches like the Government's recent awareness-raising 'See The Person' bill-board advertising campaign:

> The message behind the posters is the belief that if only society could understand the person, then disability discrimination would disappear, when in fact what is needed is fully comprehensive and enforceable civil rights legislation.
>
> (1999: 1)

Second, campaigns which concentrate solely on the reduction of disabling attitudes have, in themselves, a further disabling function:

> The Spastics Society . . . thought they were being progressive by produ-cing advertisements which encouraged people to look beyond the wheel-chair and see the real person. But if people are being asked to ignore our disability (sic) they are being asked to deny a fundamental part of our identity and our experience.
>
> (Morris, 1991: 102)

Mindful of the objections raised in the above quotations, I am aware that in seeking to increase the focus on attitudes in the social model I am entering a potential minefield, in which I could be accused of trying to sidetrack discus-sion and wider political attention away from a rightful concentration on challenging more tangible structural barriers to inclusion. Indeed, I totally agree that the almost exclusive focus on those structural barriers, and with it a concentration on the differences between disabled and non-disabled people, was justified in the early days of developing the social model, and with it a proud disabled identity which enabled many disabled people, myself included, to become more confident and to begin to challenge discrimination against us. Indeed, expressing pride in our difference remains an important statement of resistance for disabled people today. Equally, however, the logic and practical expediency of persisting with an approach which seems to assume that disabled people are always the only or the worst victims of discrimination may perhaps be questioned in a political climate which is otherwise characterized by more general philosophical developments recognizing the need to create social justice for all minorities (Phillips, 1999; Taylor, 1992), and the evidence of the growing potential to achieve this through the formation of strategic inter-group alliances for change. Such developments have been expressed in practical terms by the formation of new cross-group alliances that have come together to seek social justice. Recent examples of this collaborative approach range from small-scale local demonstrations against school closures through to the large international anti-globalization marches at economic summits.

In parallel with such wider political developments around alliance formation, mainly post-structuralist disability writers have begun to challenge assumptions of an essentialist impairment-related identity, and to suggest instead that in reality we all have multiple identities, in some of which we experience oppression, while in others we may be protected by other factors such as race, gender or class (Appleby, 1993, 1994; Corbett, 1994; Humphrey, 2000; Vernon, 1999). As will be discussed more fully in the next chapter, a multiple identity explanation may in turn create the possibility for the identification of limited common ground with non-disabled others in pursing an agenda for social change. Further, although materialist social model accounts do not adopt a multiple identities approach, some have similarly recognized the potential for change that may result from disabled people becoming involved in wider movements for social justice. For example, Finkelstein has argued that social change may best be achieved if disabled and non-disabled people start working together more systematically to tackle exclusion in all its forms (1996: 11).

However, if disabled people are to adopt this strategy, I wish to argue that we may in the process need to revisit our position on difference, and find ways of reconciling the need to preserve our identity as disabled people with the need to engage in dialogue aimed at bringing about change with others who may traditionally have had more power than us. Such an approach is potentially fraught with danger for disabled people, in that in the past those others may have used their relative power as a tool for oppression against us. It may therefore be argued by some that, if our experience is indeed wholly characterized by difference, we cannot realistically hope to find enough common ground to enable us to work as equals like this with people from other groups, and separatist political action is the only safe way forward. Yet experience suggests that disability activists have already managed to form new alliances and working partnerships with the mainstream in order to influence the development and implementation of new disability policy and practice (Campbell and Oliver, 1996; Corker, 1999: 631; Germon, 1999). Indeed, discussion of ways in which participants at Greenways similarly appeared to be able to engage through difference will be a key theme of this book. Perhaps, then, this is one area where disability theory is currently lagging behind real-world practice. It will, therefore, be suggested here that the social model has not yet fully addressed this practical need for a balancing act between preserving difference and engaging in dialogue with non-disabled others; and that more work may be needed to firm up its usefulness for activists on the ground.

Conclusion

Given the apparent limitations of any one existing explanation to explain all aspects of disabled people's experiences of inclusion and exclusion, throughout the rest of the book I have drawn on a range of sources to help explain how disability was variously constructed, replicated and challenged at Greenways Leisure Centre. Both materialist and post-structuralist social model accounts are utilized, along with normalization/SRV theory, and approaches from (mainly) post-structuralist theorists from research traditions concerned with achieving social justice for other minority groups (hooks, 2000; Giroux, 1992; Hall, 1997; Hughes, 2000; Kitzinger and Wilkinson, 1993, 1994; Mohanty, 1995; Phelan, 1995; Rattansi, 1995; Seidman, 1995; Stanley and Wise, 1993; Wilkinson and Kitzinger, 1996; Young, 1995). As a result, although the analysis that follows takes the social model as its starting point, it also draws on aspects of normalization/SRV, feminist, psychoanalytic and ethnicity theories in its attempts both to uncover some aspects of non-disabled people's constructions of disability, and to suggest some starting points in developing new alliances for change.

   In the next chapter I discuss in more detail how utilizing the concept of multiple identity helped me to analyse the complexity of the disabled/non-disabled interface, with specific reference to how my own presentation at the leisure centre as a visibly impaired person impacted on the research.

Chapter 3

Greenways Leisure Centre

Issues, identities and impairment factors

An introduction to the site

Greenways, the site where the research fieldwork was carried out, is a small community leisure centre in an industrial town in the Midlands. Leisure provision is an expanding industry in this part of the country, largely as a result of the decline of more traditional industries, and Greenways is able to draw on a large and diverse urban catchment area for its customers. Post-code research by the Centre's marketing staff indicates that most of those living in the immediate area are young people aged between 20 and 30 with small children, who are predominantly new owner-occupiers of ex-council houses, and are classified in social classes lower C and D. Marketing staff felt that this local population makes good use of the Centre, where the main facilities are a sports hall, a leisure pool with a wave machine and water slides, a lane swimming/teaching pool, a spa pool, a poolside cafe, a bar and a gymnasium. Further Centre research indicates that the site is used not only by people living close by, but also by others living within eight minutes' drive-time of the facility – a spread which in effect covers up to half the town's population. The Centre also lies on a number of bus routes, thus making it accessible to those able to use public transport.

A Centre survey of two hundred users over one month in 2000 suggested that at that time more than twice as many women than men used the Centre (approximately 70 per cent to 30 per cent), and that almost half of all users were aged 26 to 40. There were more visits in the morning (approximately 55 per cent) than in the afternoon (approximately 45 per cent), perhaps linked to independent users visiting while their children were at school. In terms of frequency of visit, the largest data group was those people using the Centre between one and three times a week. Over the period of the field-work, the day-to-day number of people using Centre facilities appeared variable, although there was a definite overall increase in visits over the time-scale of the project in 2000, from 31,000 in January to 40,000 in July. This rise coincided with the introduction of a membership scheme that offered unlimited use of all facilities upon payment of a fixed monthly fee.

In January that year there were only thirty members of this scheme, but by June over a thousand people had joined up, and as fee payment was by direct debit from people's bank accounts, there was an added incentive for them to visit regularly and hence make the most of their investment.

Throughout the project, certain time-slots at Greenways were consistently but differentially busy. For the pool it was on weekdays between 4 and 6 p.m. after school, and all day Sunday. For the gym, at least at the start of the research, the busy times tended to be from 4.30 to 8.30 p.m. on weekdays, as people stopped off there on their way home from work. However, this profile changed over time, as the new membership package resulted in an increasing number of people using the gym on a regular basis, and with more visits being reported in the daytime and at weekends. Consequently, busy and quiet periods there became more difficult to predict. Overall, researcher observation and other interview data suggest that Greenways is used primarily by 'ordinary people' of all ages looking to keep fit and enjoy their leisure, rather than by sporting champions. Observation carried out for this study, however, also suggested that the vast majority of Centre users were white. Only a very few black and Asian people were observed using the pool, with staff reporting that Asian women used another local pool instead, where it was possible to screen off the facility from view and to ensure the provision of female lifeguards for segregated sessions in a way that was not possible at Greenways. Some black teenagers (both boys and girls) did participate in indoor football and basketball tournaments held in the sports hall, but very few black and Asian people used the gym. Staff accounts for the relative absence of members of minority ethnic groups from the site are discussed in Chapter 9.

Although it was not possible to get full staffing figures for the Centre, or a breakdown of the ratio of full-time to part-time staff, or between permanent staff and those on contract, in June 2000 it appeared that there were approximately seventy-two staff in all, with a roughly equal male–female split. A strong gender imbalance was evident, however, in some specific areas of work, as discussed in more detail in Chapter 8. Five staff members (all male) were identifiably from minority ethnic groups. No figures were available on any self-declared disabled people, although one manager reported having tried in vain to persuade staff with dyslexia to declare it, so that they could receive more workplace support. It is possible to speculate that working in a setting where a 'healthy body, healthy mind' ethos was at least sometimes in evidence might have made staff reluctant to reveal any perceived personal deviation from the norm. Another staffing factor that proved especially important in terms of this research was that, in addition to the permanent and contract staff based permanently at the Centre, a number of external contractors were also used to teach particular classes – including all those I observed which were offered specifically to disabled people. This gave me the opportunity to compare the approaches to inclusion offered by external staff with those of the Centre's own workforce, and to explore the relative impact of Greenways' equalities policies on those internal and external staff – a comparison which showed up some worrying differences in the quality of service provision on offer to disabled customers. I will elaborate on these findings in more detail later in the book.

The period of time chosen for the study proved (accidentally) to be a particularly interesting one, because it coincided with the transition of the organization from the public to the private sector, as it took on trust status. In operational terms, this move resulted in a change of emphasis from leisure provision at any cost, to a focus on debt reduction and income generation; whilst in human terms it was a time of potentially unsettling change, requiring staff to adopt new business-oriented ways of working which focused not only on customer service but on income generation as well. Not all staff were able or willing to make this transition, and a number of them left – or were eased out – during the period of the study. These changes came about within the wider context of increasing competition in leisure provision in the area, and stemmed from a perceived need to compete with the private sector, and in so doing to reduce the amount of debt still owing to the local authority as a result of the original high Centre building costs. As became apparent from discussions with a range of staff, however, tensions existed within the organization around its future direction and priorities, with some staff actively embracing the new 'empowerment culture' and the move to attract new customers with greater amounts of disposable income, and others expressing concern at the possible resulting emergence of a two-tier service.

This general tension was reflected in the range of reactions expressed towards the new membership scheme. Although the massive growth in membership represented a welcome growth in income, and was also widely agreed to represent a good deal for customers, the scheme was seen as somewhat problematic because it operated on a direct debit basis, and hence was only open to people who held bank accounts and who could in addition afford to make regular monthly payments. Even staff committed to the scheme recognized that these conditions excluded a range of poor people, and others such as some older people in the area who historically and culturally preferred not to have bank accounts. Instead, these groups had no option but to continue to use the old pay-as-you-go system inherited from the local authority management days. In addition, anecdotal evidence suggested that the increase in members wanting to use parts of the facility, particularly the gym, had led on occasion to their needs being prioritized over those of the pay-as-you-go customers. It was felt that this trend was likely to be reinforced with the planned future refurbishment of the Centre, with some of the new upgraded facilities being reserved for members only. Thus at least some of the staff were already aware that structural factors to do with service provision could have a real impact on customer experience of inclusion and exclusion at the site.

However, despite the move towards a more business-oriented approach, the Centre retained a strong community ethos. There were clear attempts to retain elements of 'the organization as a family' that had previously been a strong feature of service provision, and the new marketing strategies continued to be based around valuing the audience over the product. Regular customers were included as part of the Centre scene, there were barbeques and evenings out at local nightclubs organized by the gym staff, and during the fieldwork there was frequent evidence of staff stopping for social chats with users. In addition, the presence of an enthusiastic, committed community development officer ensured the provision of a con-tinuing (often loss-making) service to a range of 'minority groups', such as older people, disabled people, young black footballers, mums and babies, a local church congregation, and people on a low income. However, most of this provision was segregated and staffed by external contractors, and took place at times when the Centre would otherwise be underused. For some groups this presented a problem, and they reported that their inconvenient time-slot made it difficult for them to recruit quality coaching staff. Such issues demonstrate the increasingly difficult balancing act in activity programming faced by Centre managers between the need to maximize income while continuing to prove a service to all sectors of the community (Torkildsen, 1993: 6.03). Still, the need for social provision remained impor-tant to the Centre's ethos, as demonstrated by the fact that the community liaison role was not restricted solely to the named community development officer. Other service-based initiatives included negotiation by the marketing department of free media publicity on behalf of local sports groups, in the hope that this would extend existing community links; the existence of strong connections between the leisure centre and the town's medical services, with some sessions being organized specifically for people referred for exercise regimes by their doctors; and a general public commitment to anti-discrimination practices at the site, expressed through wall posters located in prominent places around the building. Thus the Centre retained a strong ongoing commitment to providing a service to the local community, even though it was experiencing increasing pressure to focus on commercial goals.

Having thus set the scene by describing some of the issues that already had an effect on staff relationships and service provision at Greenways, the remainder of this chapter discusses some of the identity-related and personal issues that influenced the way in which I conducted the research.

Multiple identity as a tool for understanding disability construction

When I first started planning the fieldwork element of the project, I struggled both to make a choice about which of my identities should be primary when I went to Greenways, and to find strategies which might enable me to avoid my presence as a disabled person having an undue influence on events, in case my subsequent research findings were dismissed as being 'too subjective' because of my impairment status. Very early on, however, I realized that in making decisions about how to conduct the research I could not avoid drawing on my wider life experience, in which I have been lucky enough to have formed rich personal and working relationships with people from diverse backgrounds and beliefs. I knew that at least some of these interactions and connections would not have been possible had my own belief system been incapable of movement through persuasion by others, or if those others with whom I was making connections had assimilated wholesale the binary notion of difference, where that difference is only attributed to the person with minority status. Instead, it was in part our understanding that actually we were different from each other (Phelan, 1995: 334) that made the connection work. Even though we were not equally oppressed all of the time, we recognized that we had all experienced some struggles, and that 'we had a greater unity when people focused truthfully on their own experiences' rather than worrying that they 'were irrelevant because they were not as oppressive or as exploited as the experiences of others' (hooks, 2000: 59).

Given this life experience, I realized it would be difficult for me to adopt an essentialist position in this research. In other words, I did not want to explore my relationships with other people purely in terms of our relative impairment status. Instead, I wanted to be open to the possibility that other factors associated with my identity might affect how people reacted around me. In turn, I hoped that uncovering additional routes of communication in this way might offer some potential for making connections and new alliances for change with previously unconsidered others. Thus in conducting the research I hoped to test out whether, and if so to what extent, adopting a multiple identity approach was indeed an appropriate and achievable strategy to promote social change. This sort of pluralist approach made sense to me, even as I acknowledged the counter-arguments against it (Erevelles, 1996). At a personal level I could see the dangers of an approach which, in acknowledging the value of alliances with people who were not 'like me', risked the dilution or outright loss of aspects of my core identity, in particular my self-image as a proud disabled person. Further, as has previously been argued, a strategy of multiple identification can lead to an infinite regression into only looking at individuals (Young, 1995: 195), thereby losing a sense of group identity and broad group political strategy, and also obscuring the individual's relative investments in particular identities (Rattansi, 1995: 271). And in campaigning for wider change, the risk also remains of disabled people's needs (as so often in the past) being overlooked or pushed to the end of the queue in favour of those with louder voices (Young, 1995: 197). So, yes, pluralism and coalitions as advocated by disability theorists and activists alike (Appleby, 1994; Corbett, 1994; Humphrey, 1999; Vernon, 1999) are not unproblematic strategies. And yet, the longer I spent in the field, and the more contacts I made there, the less sure I became that any one epistemological standpoint could help me to explain what I was seeing, and the more I learned through talking to people at the site about the potential which could be unleashed through the making of new alliances (Giroux, 1992: 26; Rattansi, 1995: 278–80), including those with members of the so-called mainstream. In practical terms, too, I wanted to test out whether the development of situationally appropriate coalitions might offer the potential to avoid the problems of despair and burn-out which can affect all activists who attempt to challenge the existing order (GMCDP, 2000; Phelan, 1995: 349).

In pursuing a pluralist approach, the research shares some concerns with Mohanty (1995: 78–9), who believes that social movements and their related theories and identity politics may nurture their members for a while, but can 'ultimately provide an illusion of community based on isolation and the freezing of difference'. In her view, it isn't the experience of, for example, being a woman which is important, but 'the meanings attached to gender, race, class, and age at various historical moments that is of strategic significance'. Hence the fact of being a woman, or being a disabled person, isn't in itself the key – it's about where the core of power lies in each case. Thus for her, the way forward in terms of achieving feminist political change is for members from a range of minority groups to share their experience and understanding of oppression as the next step towards challenging it:

> Instead of privileging a certain limited version of identity politics, it is the current *intersection* of antiracist, anti-imperialist, and gay and lesbian struggles which we need to understand to map the ground for feminist political strategy and political analysis.
>
> (ibid.: 81)

In practical terms, this suggests for all minorities the possibility of forming coalitions with other groups to tackle a range of issues, just as Finkelstein (1996: 11) has specifically called upon the disability movement to do. Similarly Finger (1991: 43), in acknowledging that bringing up a disabled child may mean extra work for the mother, suggests that 'we could link our struggles for women, for disabled people, working together for better social services, disability rights legislation, working for more equitable distribution of work within families, instead of seeing our interests as unalterably opposed'. And Phelan (1995: 341) has argued that although the goal of decent housing is a lesbian issue, poor housing also affects many other people. Lesbians may encounter particular problems about being 'out' in the community in poor neighbourhoods, but this also ties in with the wider problem of how to get decent housing on a low income. So, whilst acknowledging that there may be specific differences between the experiences of poor lesbians and poor straight people, there are also some areas of commonality. She believes, therefore, that in this situation it would be possible to establish a limited common agenda between all the people struggling against poor housing, without succumbing to the dangers of either essentialism or of overgeneralization.

Some dangers of self-revelation for minority researchers

Even after I had decided on a multiple identity approach, however, for a long time I still retained a strong preference against any revelation of 'my self' in the presentation of the data. This decision stemmed from earlier life experiences of being held up as a 'role model' for other disabled people, a position which had only served to damage both myself and those others. Hence I have always been in total solidarity with the disabled people's movement in its rage against the portrayal of the 'super-crip', those illusory disabled people who are presented in the media as having 'overcome their handicaps' and achieved superhuman feats of courage or endurance. Such images have, in reality, been created by non-disabled people to reassure themselves and to lessen their fear of impairment and of the loss of bodily control represented by ordinary disabled people (Morris, 1991: 101), and have done little or nothing to promote social inclusion for the mass of disabled people on our own terms.

I was also acutely aware of the disapproval of many materialist social model theorists, notably Finkelstein (1996: 11), of disability research which concentrates on reporting individual experience without reference to the wider context of social oppression and structural barriers which are faced by disabled people as a group (Thomas, 1999: 75), and was anxious to avoid any such charge of narcissism in my own work. In fact, however, such problems of representation and analysis are not restricted solely to the disability movement. Giroux (1992: 80) reports bell hooks' warning of the same dangers for feminism in reporting individual experience without situating it within wider theoretical and critical analysis. However, when I started out on this project it did not seem possible that, in disclosing anything of my own experience in the field, I could avoid falling into just such a trap. In addition, all the time that I remained in pursuit of the goal of being a neutral researcher, I was loath to concede that in any way I might only be able to collect the fieldwork data because of who I am. It felt like going against two orthodoxies here: that of the disabled people's movement, part of which objects to the presentation of individual disabled people's subjective experience as a way of helping to make sense of our oppression (Finkelstein, 1996: 11); and that of academia in its preference for the researcher to be a neutral and 'objective' reporter of events in the field (Cohen and Manion, 1994; Hammersley, 1998; Hammersley and Atkinson, 1983). So how would these political and methodological principles square with my choice of a topic of study in which I had many personal investments outside the research framework? Would anything I wrote about non-disabled people's constructions of disability be seen as 'too subjective', because too much implicated with my own life experience? For a long time, struggling with these issues made it difficult to move the project forward in any meaningful way.

Embracing the inevitability of the 'researcher effect'

And yet, the more I fought against owning my personal investments in the project as a disabled person, the more I had started to read about fieldwork strategies which recognized the inevitability of the 'researcher effect' on the field of study (Clough, 1996; Coffey, 1999; Fine, 1994; Ozga and Gewirtz, 1994; Sparkes, 1994, 1995, 1996; Stanley and Wise, 1993). The more, too, I was finding myself in the fieldwork itself drawing on my previous experience as a consultant and trainer, and as someone who had gone through a process of organizational change similar to that being experienced by Greenways staff at the time of the research. Clearly, then, my identity as a disabled person was not the only one I was using here – it was not the only one that made sense to me at all times. And at this point I realized that I had to acknowledge, and make explicit, the whole range of identities I occupied in the field, and how that mix had enabled me to collect the data for the project.

Thus in developing good-enough working relationships with staff and users at Greenways, I found myself drawing on a whole range of previous experiences. Having understood for much of my life that many people will never be able to connect first off with the whole of me, I utilized the knowledge of that unpalatable truth in developing the project. My fieldwork strategy thus became one of deconstructing myself, as a first step towards showing people that perhaps there were selected bits of me that they could relate to, even if they couldn't deal with all of me at once. And if they could do it with me, perhaps that would give them the confidence in future to do the same with other people new to them. The process of making explicit this deconstruction also seemed to open up new possibilities for me at a personal level. In examining and reshaping some of my previously assumed identities and subjectivities (Phelan, 1995: 345), I began to learn to be proud of the whole complex jumble of who I am, rather than pretending that the academic part of me was the only bit which was important now.

When it came to analysing the data, I discovered that I had accumulated a diverse range of material – from examples of wholly inclusive practice through to ones of downright abuse – and realized that I needed to find a framework which could help me work out how this had come about. Eventually I came to understand that what people in the field had chosen to reveal to me was largely dependent on who they thought I was at the time of our interaction. Hence, for example, those engaged in apparent abuse seemingly had no hesitation in letting me see what they were doing, because even though I had told them that I was a researcher, they could only see me as someone who was in their eyes a relatively powerless disabled person, and that as such they expected me to collude with them by my silence.

Once I had understood that this process of identity assignment was taking place, it seemed only logical to analyse and present the project data through a series of chapters, each one based on an aspect of my identity in the field. In turn, each shows people's varying constructions of disability, and how these shifted depending on which aspect of my identity they were relating to at that time. In total over the course of the fieldwork I identified the following research identities: researcher, consultant, member of staff, friend, woman, white person, embodied being, disabled person, oppressor and activist. That's ten in all, and excludes the more nebulous aspect of the equation of my 'personality', which has proved more difficult to report on. Using the concept of identity as the organizing principle in this way also helped to overcome my dilemma about explaining why the research 'worked' for me. Actually it worked – or not – in different ways in different situations, depending on which identities both I and the other parties chose to be primary at that time, and of course those identities could then change again even in the course of the conversation.

In using this analytical approach to understanding the research data, I was influenced in part by Mouffe (1995: 317–18). In discussing strategies for feminist movement, she has said that, while some people argue that deconstruction of essential identities makes feminist political action impossible, she thinks it is necessary for an 'adequate understanding of the variety of social relations where the principles of liberty and equality should apply'. In practical terms, therefore, she argues that we need to lose the idea of a rational subject and of unified positions in order to 'theorize the multiplicity of relations of subordination', where the same person may be 'dominant in one relation while subordinated in another'. In this particular research setting, the dimensions of time, space and relationality also contributed to destabilizing any sense of myself as an essentialist, unified whole (Somers, 1994: 606). A deconstructionist approach to reporting my research findings therefore came to make particular explanatory sense to me, since it was clear during the fieldwork that I was not consistently either powerful or powerless throughout, but experienced a range of positions depending upon whom I was talking to, and in what role or context. In retrospect, I suspect that the process of making these decisions about who I was in the field, and how to present the complex and sometimes contradictory data collected, probably marks the point where I moved beyond the binary in this work.

Impairment factors: strategies for self-presentation in the field

Choosing to conduct research in a leisure setting also had some very personal implications for me. In particular, working in a place where people went to exercise and keep fit meant that it would have been extremely difficult to divorce the intellectual work from the reality of my own embodiment, even if I had wanted to do so. As a result, before starting the fieldwork it was necessary to make a number of decisions about my self-presentation in the setting. In order to blend into the background as far as possible I opted for casual dress, usually wearing tracksuit bottoms and a t-shirt, but with the precautionary extra of a fleece when observing action in the sports hall, which throughout the winter and spring was very cold. As such I usually seemed to pass as an ordinary user. Being in a leisure setting also made it easy to observe many of the activities on offer, especially in the pool and the sports hall, because often I was only one of a number of spectators there, and as such I did not look out of place.

However, there were a number of additional factors around self-representation arising specifically out of my impairment, about which I had to think and make decisions. In general I have noticed that previously few disability researchers have been particularly explicit about the additional impairment-related factors they have to take account of in carrying out their work, a recent exception being described in Paterson and Hughes (1999). However, in choosing to focus here on people's constructions of disability, I could not ignore the potential impact of my own embodiment on the research process. Nor did I want to pretend that in tackling such a sensitive issue there were no personal risks for me. Later chapters will discuss how I dealt with some of the difficult personal issues that arose in the course of the research. For now, I want to describe the process I went through in deciding how to present myself in this setting as someone with a visible impairment (cerebral palsy), and what problems and opportunities that led to in conducting the research. In doing so, I hope to show that it is not always necessary for disabled researchers to underplay in public arenas the realities of their impairments and their potential effect on the research process, simply because convention and mainstream prejudice dictates that we should do so.

Initially, at the most basic level, I had to decide whether to present myself at Greenways as a wheelchair user, or as an ambulant mobility-impaired person. My original preference, for a number of reasons, was to go in as ambulant. Since beginning a few years ago to use a wheelchair some of the time, I had been struck by the general improvement in people's reactions to me, and the increase in levels of unsolicited support on offer. When I used to walk all the time, especially before I started using a stick, I found most people acted at best as if I was not there, and at worst as if I was a drunk who deserved all I got. If I was walking down the street I would often end up walking twice as far as everyone else, simply because people would not give any ground on the pavement, or because they just did not want to acknowledge my presence and were instead desperately trying to pretend that I wasn't there. Either way, I usually had to escape into the gutter to avoid being knocked over. I also noticed that people found it particularly hard back then to deal with my speech impairment, especially if they met me when I was sitting down, and hence had no prior warning of any potential bodily differences. When my speech impairment kicked in they would go red, look away or sometimes even walk off, leaving me in mid-sentence. None of this was calculated to enhance my self-esteem.

Since I started using a chair, however, things have definitely changed for the better, although I suspect this has come about for all the wrong reasons. Nowadays people move out of my way in the street, though mainly because I think they realize that they would come off worse than me in a collision. And I experience far fewer negative reactions to my speech than before, but I suspect this is because to many non-disabled people the wheelchair is still a universal signifier of incompetence, and hence that they see any additional differences or 'unusual behaviour' as being simply to be expected. At a political level, I find it outrageous that such stereotypes apparently retain a strong hold on the public consciousness. At the same time, however, at a personal level I have to admit that my life is much easier and less stressful as a result. This is just one example of how much easier it is to collude with existing power relations than it is to suggest that we look for ways to move beyond them (Giroux, 1992), when those new ways are likely to require more personal effort to make them succeed.

On balance then, I felt that the project would be more likely to uncover extremes of negative behaviour if I presented as ambulant. However, other factors militated against this. With fatigue and pain becoming increasing personal issues, I had to be realistic and ask myself if I would really be able to undertake extended periods of fieldwork standing up, and having to be able to carry notebooks, tape recorder, and so on and use my stick at the same time. Then too, there was the issue of having to negotiate a range of surfaces, some of which would be wet. I realized it might prove difficult to observe what was going on around me if all my attention and energy had to go on watching where to put my feet, and on avoiding people who

were about to walk into me. And so I was reluctantly drawn to the conclusion that it would be easier all round to present as a wheelchair user.
However, in selecting this presentation strategy, I must reiterate my suspicion
that I would have been far more likely to have uncovered the existence of a
wider range of disablist oppression towards me as an individual had I been
able to go into this setting as an ambulant disabled person.

Entering a sports setting as a wheelchair user was in itself not entirely
unproblematic. Until then I had only used my chair on an occasional basis,
and usually with a support worker on hand to bale me out if I got tired
or lost control of speed or direction. The prospect of now attempting to
present myself at Greenways as a routine and competent wheelchair user
when actually I wasn't sure if I had the necessary technical skills to do so
was quite daunting, especially when I ran over somebody's foot during my
first site visit. At that point I would have been delighted if the ground had
opened and swallowed me up. And then, too, there was the more general
issue to be dealt with of how I myself felt about being seen as a wheelchair
user, when I had spent so many years and so much energy trying to stay
on my feet. Internalized oppression had done a good job on me in making
me feel that in some massive way using a chair represented failure. And
there was the influence of sheer vanity to contend with, too. I really did
not want James, my main contact at Greenways, whom I already knew to
be a leading sportsman in his own right who makes regular appearances in
the media, to see me as a wheelchair user. Looking back, I'm not sure who
I was trying to kid here – whether I present as a wheelchair user or as
ambulant, I am never going to be mistaken for a non-disabled person. But
I guess acknowledging that takes some time.

In any case, I ended up using my chair for most of the fieldwork, and on
balance this was definitely the most sensible course of action. It also
appeared to open up new possibilities for conducting the research. For
example, my chair has detachable handles, and often I choose not to put
them on, having had my fair share of perfect strangers coming up to me in
public places, grabbing the handles without first asking my permission,
and taking me (usually at high speed) somewhere I didn't want to go.
Now, at Greenways, I took the conscious decision at the start of each visit
to add the handles, to see what would happen in this setting. I was particularly interested to find out whether people's behaviour would change over
time, and whether they might become more or less respectful of my private
space as they got used to me being around.

As a relative wheelchair novice, I initially had no intention of taking
part in any sports activities on offer, and felt that being detached from the
general sports and leisure ethos in this way would give me the opportunity
to act almost as an anthropologist, observing and trying to make sense of
events from an outsider perspective. However, in the event such detachment
was not possible, for a number of reasons. First, most users of the leisure

centre turned out to be ordinary unpretentious individuals, seemingly more interested in maintaining their existing fitness levels, or in losing weight before going on holiday, than in becoming Mr or Ms Universe. Thus in fact it turned out that we weren't all that different from each other after all. Second, it was not long before I realized that being in the setting was reawakening my own former sporting impulses, which I thought I had successfully dampened down during a long period of illness. Now it became clear that, despite my best efforts, my competitive streak was still alive and kicking, making a wholly disinterested approach to participation difficult to maintain. Third, although it was perfectly possible to sit and watch events in the pool and the sports hall, the same was not true of the gym, as I found on my first access negotiation visit. Users there appeared extremely uncomfortable at having me watching them, and it was the first time in ages that I actually felt waves of hatred coming my way. The situation probably wasn't helped either in that I had been accompanied that day by James. It is very hard to read off that original gym visit, and the user reactions, at any one level. Was it that they objected to being watched by a smartly dressed woman and a man in a suit while they were hot and sweaty in their work-out gear? Was it that we, as a black man and a disabled woman, were the ones doing the watching for once, rather than vice versa? Did they feel particularly exposed at being watched by him as a nationally recognized athlete? Or would they have reacted just as negatively had we both been white, be-suited, middle-class men?

Even now, I still can't explain exactly why we attracted such hostility that day, but the experience did point up just how difficult it would be to pin any one explanation on events in the field. It also made me realize that I would not be able to use observation techniques in the gym, unless I wanted to risk getting lynched. It would have to be participation, or nothing. Hence, within a couple of weeks of starting the fieldwork, I knew that I would have to become a more active participant in the setting, if I was to engender trust among other users. It was at this point that any illusions I had started out with of being able to act as a neutral researcher in this setting finally disappeared.

Chapter 4

Being a researcher

Dilemmas about how to collect the data

In seeking to study the interface between disabled and non-disabled people I found myself using an unconventional research approach, not only as a member of a minority group studying the behaviour of a majority, but also in terms of the range of methodologies and methods that I drew on in doing so. In deciding which approaches to use I wanted, for example, to challenge the commonsense assumption that it was neither possible nor appropriate to use 'participatory' research techniques as defined/adopted by disabled people (Zarb, 1992), in conducting disability research with non-disabled people. I was aware that participatory research approaches had been used before in studying various aspects of non-disabled people's experience as a way of giving some control over the research process to those being studied (Hammersley, 1998: 16), but hadn't previously come across it in cases like this one where the research was disability-related and the researcher was a disabled person. In fact I realized that I didn't really have an existing research template to follow, and that I might have to try out a range of strategies in order to collect the research data. However, I still wanted to try a broadly participatory approach. An important reason for this was that the research aimed to explore the possibilities for making some connections between disabled and non-disabled people's experiences, and as such I knew that some of the issues under discussion might prove to be sensitive ground for the participants. In these circumstances, I thought it was important to be as respectful as possible of their needs, and in so doing to lessen the chances that they would feel unreasonably exploited by the research process. I felt that a participatory approach offered the potential to achieve this aim.

Early informal exploration of my research topic with various disability studies researchers, however, suggested a specific objection to the use of participatory research techniques with non-disabled people in this study, on the grounds that such an approach would keep existing power relations intact. To a certain extent I could understand this concern. Both as a disabled person, and as a woman, I was initially worried that any attempt to share ownership of the research process with non-disabled subjects would mean that I could lose control of my research. However, I was concerned to explore this objection, and wished to test out the proposition that it is only by attempting to find ways of engaging on equal terms with non-disabled people that the profile of existing power relations can be properly mapped out, as a first step towards then challenging them. I remain aware that some people have still found my approach either foolhardy or diversionary. However, in going ahead with it I was deliberately experimenting with the possibilities that might be generated. In doing so I also had to confront my distrust of unfamiliar non-disabled people, and to hope that they would 'play by the rules' in the same way that disabled people have when I've inter-viewed them in the past, rather than attempting to hijack the research for their own ends. This is not to say that at the outset I was not scared at what might happen when I tried to apply these principles in the cold reality of the fieldwork setting – I was! On top of everything else, then, this decision-making process was also an early indication of the ongoing diffi-culty I found in trying to separate out different aspects of the research experi-ence. Here, my identities as researcher, disabled person and woman were all directly implicated in the decisions I made about how to conduct the research.

Following on from this point, a more general concern about my role in researching non-disabled people came up in the suggestion that it might not be possible for me as a disabled person to interview non-disabled people direct, especially about their attitudes towards disabled people, because they wouldn't tell me 'the truth'. Inevitably, in this study my presence and role as a disabled person did have an effect on the research process (Connolly, 1996: 195). However, it may be argued that researcher effect is potentially an issue in all interviewing, where it is hard to be sure that the subject is not just telling you what they think you want to hear (Henwood and Pidgeon, 1993: 24; Silverman, 1993: 100). Even when the subject is telling you the truth as they see it, it will only ever be a situationally appropriate partial account based on one version or story of what the truth is (Silverman, 1993: 95). And, then, as another researcher from a minority background said:

> Why can't you interview them about disability? They may say things that you don't want to hear, or on the other hand they may attempt a politically correct response, but you're going to know when they're faking it.

This challenge made me decide to go ahead, although I remained aware that there were potential dangers in my trying to analyse the data based on its relations to my personal experience, and on my own assumptions about the reasons why people behave in particular ways.

Ethical issues

The other big issue around my decision to conduct research with non-disabled people was an ethical one. In particular I needed to be clear about how honest I should be with the participants about the real purpose of my research, and was especially mindful of Ozga and Gewirtz's comment (1994: 129) that it is a mistake to think that members of elite groups (here, non-disabled people) are not 'vulnerable to exploitation or misrepresentation'. However, my primary concern was that if I told participants upfront that I was there to study their constructions of disability, they might indeed change their behaviour and just tell me what they thought I wanted to hear. I discussed this dilemma with James, my main contact and gatekeeper of access to the site, who as a black man used to facing negative attitudes understood the potential problem here. I was completely honest with him about my research aims, but we agreed that to be equally transparent with the other participants might affect their behaviour and make the research meaningless. As a result, in my early contact with them I deliberately adopted a cover story to explain my presence which made no mention of my real interest in studying their constructions of disability, and which instead suggested that my remit was to look at the way the organization worked, and at community use of Centre facilities (in fact this was indeed part of what I did – but only one part). More direct questioning about disability issues only took place later, once they had become more used to my presence on site. Following Gillborn's approach (1990: 210) in his study of race, ethnicity and education, I was also careful to avoid being the first one to talk about disability and impairment during our conversations, so as to minimize the possibility of bias or of being seen to unduly influence what they talked about.

Despite adopting such strategies, however, I found that within weeks of my arrival most members of Greenways' staff had made the assumption anyway that I was there primarily to work with disabled customers. This suggested both that at the outset my identity as a disabled person was the one they automatically engaged with first, and also that they could not imagine that I might actually be there to study them as the majority group of non-disabled people. In fact I was able to use this second assumption to my advantage, especially during the early stages of the research when I was still a relatively unknown quantity for them, because it meant that I was often able to observe their interactions unchallenged, and that they remained largely unselfconscious in my presence. However, by not being more open about my motives from the outset, I am aware that I could be accused of dishonesty in my approach, although perhaps no more so than any other ethnographic 'under-cover' researcher. In fact, as the research progressed, both my liking for and sense of responsibility towards the participants grew, and I found myself putting some of my technical skills at their disposal, as discussed in Chapter 5. At least part of the reason for this arose from my sense of guilt at having misled them at the outset in this way.

Power relations in the research process

Overall, I was amazed at the innocence of the research process demonstrated by the non-disabled participants, and especially among those members of staff whom I formally interviewed as part of the project. In particular, they seemed completely unaware of the potential for abuse of power by the researcher that I had been so concerned about at the beginning of the field-work. For example, none appeared concerned that I might repeat what they had told me to the management, or use the data to misrepresent their views, or sell their stories to the press. This high level of trust was in sharp contrast to my previous experience of working with disabled people. In addition, several participants were keen for their own identities, and for that of the Centre, to be made public, a request which of course went against the code of research confidentiality. Some indeed seemed to feel that such publicity was their due reward for talking to me, and were quite disappointed when I explained that I couldn't do it. It certainly made me wonder about how much they felt valued at Greenways, that they were looking to me as an outsider to publicize and thus, by implication in their eyes, to vindicate their views.

In fact, the formal interview phase of the research proved to be especially useful in uncovering some subtle aspects of disabled/non-disabled power relations that observation and participation alone might not have revealed. To begin with, in terms of what people said at interview, I decided that I would not question any use of inappropriate or disabling terminology on their part, since one of the purposes of the research was to report where people are now, rather than to challenge overtly what they said. I was afraid that if I did question their use of language it might make them so uncomfortable or defensive that they would clam up altogether. At times I found this strategy hard to maintain, because it was at odds with my desire as an action researcher and activist to bring about positive change in the setting. However, I persevered with it, even when the outcome was personally depressing. Use of outdated terms and phrases such as 'the disabled', 'the mentally handicapped', and 'confined to a wheelchair' was common across interviewees of all ages, and some of the opinions expressed were of a paternalistic nature, based on an expectation that most disabled people needed 'looking after' and were best served in that setting by segregated leisure provision. Precisely whom they meant by 'disabled people' here is discussed in more detail in Chapter 11. For now the main point to be made is that my interview strategy seemed to work, in that people did appear to feel free to express their real views, with little apparent attempt at politically correct responses. Either that, or they were genuinely unaware of how inappropriate some of their comments were.

In some cases participants displayed a mixture of disablism and awareness, sometimes even within individual statements, as in the following extract, where one person is talking about their previous experience of working with disabled people:

> they were really severely handicapped. But I suppose, I didn't work with them too long, but it's a funny thing – you get attached, even so you get attached, don't you? You get to know their funny mannerisms and that. But there again, I take people as I see them. It's not a thing I worry about. It wouldn't scare me. Yet some people are scared, aren't they?

The first part of this comment in particular is deeply offensive and patronizing. Yet towards the end the interviewee makes a valid point about non-disabled people's fear of difference affecting how they act. At one level as a disabled person I do not want to have to engage with people who use such inappropriate language, imbued with negative value judgements about disabled people as 'the other'. There are undoubtedly times in my personal life when I know I would not be prepared to make the effort needed to talk to someone like that, when we seem to be coming at the world from such different angles. However, in this setting I felt that I had a responsibility as a researcher to where possible put my own feelings to one side and to concentrate on the academic exercise of charting existing constructions of disability, as a first step to developing wider strategies to change them. Such an approach sometimes brought unexpected rewards, as when later in the same interview this person made one of the most logical arguments on the benefits of disabled and non-disabled people working together that I have ever come across (see Chapter 9). This showed that it was simply not possible to dismiss everything that some people said simply because of the way they said it. However, such examples also reinforce the point that making alliances with non-disabled people may not always be easy.

From the data collected, it was not possible to demonstrate any real differences in disability construction based on interviewee gender, although in some cases the approach to achieving inclusion seemed for some women to be based more on increasing empathy and developing a general understanding of disabled people's needs, while for some men a targeted problem-solving approach to specific identified barriers was preferred. Certainly the data collected added force to my subsequent recommendation to management that disability equality training be given to all staff, to improve both their general awareness of disability issues and their customer service provision.

In part I suspect that the staff members' relative openness in what they told me during the research was because most of our formal interview discussions were 'about' their work identities rather than their personal ones, so I was not asking them to share anything private or unduly sensitive. Also, of course, there was more than one set of power relations at work here – the researcher–researched, the staff member–outsider, and perhaps also the non-disabled–disabled difference (though in many cases it felt like we moved beyond this one). However they were 'reading' me in each case, it was certainly true that power did not automatically and constantly reside with either of us throughout the interview. For example, one person reported being frightened of being asked to take part, while another, having initially agreed to it, then tried to avoid coming along. Some participants automatically and without comment set up the tape recorder and turned the pages of my notes for me as we went along. One person even took the interview sheet from me, and proceeded to ask himself the questions. I found this particular behaviour a bit bizarre, until I reflected that the powerlessness which I was now feeling was probably indicative of what he himself felt, either about the interview situation in particular or his wider role at the Centre. This observation was particularly relevant because I knew he was about to leave the organization. Once I had realized there was more than one possible explanation for his behaviour, I was then able to relax and go along with it, and as a result collected some useful data. More difficult to deal with were those very few interviewees who constantly interrupted or talked over the top of me. In those cases I found it hard to contain my anger at their rudeness, and sometimes found myself becoming increasingly inattentive, as though I could not be bothered to listen to them if they wouldn't extend the same courtesy to me. Fortunately having the tape recorder on meant that I could still provide them with an accurate transcript afterwards, once I'd calmed down enough to trust myself to write it up.

Power relations here compared with those implicated in research with disabled people

One of the findings of this research which I struggled for some months to understand was how little importance any of the interview participants attached to their interview transcript. When I have negotiated interviews with disabled people in the past, the provision of a verbatim transcript has usually been one of their preconditions for taking part. Here, though, there appeared to be no such imperative. Few people gave any feedback on what I'd written, or asked for text to be removed or changed, except where the use of expletives or dialect was involved and the participants were concerned that keeping these words in would make them sound rude or stupid. In such cases I had no hesitation in removing the offending text, just as I did not reproduce the effects of my stammer, because I realized that actually what we were saying to each other was far more important than how we were saying it. This one issue of representation apart, none of the participants seemed to attach the same value to the transcripts as they had done to the actual interviews. I even came across one transcript that had been left in an unlocked filing cabinet where anyone could have found and read it. These responses led me to think that I was more concerned about respecting interviewee confidentiality than the participants themselves were. I didn't know what to make of this at all, because it contrasted so sharply with my previous research experience with disabled people. At one point I was so confused that I even asked James why he thought people were so laid back about it, but he just looked nonplussed at the question, so I was left none the wiser. Looking back on it now I think their response was partly due to the fact, as suggested above, that during the interviews we had been discussing their public work lives, whereas with disabled people the research topic is often more personal and private so they would naturally be especially concerned to ensure that they retained some control over what went out into the public domain. Then again, another researcher suggested it might just have been that the staff at Greenways trusted me. If so, I find this horrifying. I know from personal experience of research exploitation that I would never automatically trust another researcher to represent my views without instigating some sort of power to discuss the raw data, or in extreme cases to veto publication of what they wrote about me.

Eventually it was Sinason's analysis (1992: 202–4) of the importance of the scribe function for disabled people which – paradoxically – provided me with a fuller explanation of what was going on at Greenways. She explains how, for disabled people who experience loss of physical function or who have learning difficulties, it may be difficult or impossible for them to tell their own stories independently without the physical input provided by a scribe. Hence the involvement of that scribe means that for the disabled person 'an experience is being offered of healthy omnipotence' which might otherwise be unavailable to her. For some disabled people, then, the interview experience may provide a unique opportunity to voice feelings, thoughts and emotions that they have never had the chance to express before. Further, owning the resultant interview transcript may be one of the few occasions where their words have been valued and their history written down in their own terms. Certainly this tied in with my own experience during a previous research project I conducted with disabled women. On that occasion (Tregaskis, 1998), all the interviewees told me that 'Nobody has ever asked me about this part of my life before', and all had welcomed receipt of their transcripts. Conversely, with these non-disabled participants, I came to realize that, quite simply, they had no need of a scribe to make public their thoughts and feelings. They were not at the same risk as many disabled people are of having their views remaining in their own heads and unacknowledged by the world; and that was why their interview transcripts did not hold the same significance for them.

It was also significant that although James was a black man facing daily oppression, he too did not have the same need of a transcript as did the disabled people I had worked with previously. As I now realized, despite his experience of oppression he could still write and speak his own account, and find ways of processing his thoughts and of having them believed, because he was both a senior manager at Greenways and a sporting celebrity, and thus was relatively powerful. Some disability experience, on the other hand, makes disabled people so powerless that they effectively have no voice, and/or may face enormous physical, mental and emotional barriers to telling their own stories. These barriers are qualitatively greater than those faced by most non-disabled people. This, then, is one area of the research process where I truly feel that the experience of disabled people is different, even from that of other acknowledged minority groups. I am not sure, however, that the significance of this aspect of power relations is always fully acknowledged or understood by researchers, thus leaving open the possibility of (often unwitting) abuse of disabled participants. I believe, therefore, that all disability researchers need to understand that, where enough trust is engendered with disabled people that they agree to share their experiences, then that researcher has to accept that they in turn are implicated in helping to make sense of what has happened in the disabled person's life. Even if this is achieved only by believing them enough to put in the time and effort to record a full transcript, and ensuring that ownership of that data remains with the disabled person, this is still an important starting point in beginning to reduce unequal power relations.

For my own part, untangling this part of the power relations at Greenways also provided a valuable lesson by showing me that some aspects of participatory research may have greater or lesser significance for particular groups being researched. I came to realize that there are some aspects of people's lived experience within society which *are* different. Many disabled people are effectively without a voice or have it misinterpreted by the wider world, whereas the non-disabled people being studied here clearly felt at no risk from the research process (or at least, at that which was personified by me as a disabled, female researcher). In summary, then, the 'one model fits all' research approach which I had tried to adopt at the outset proved in practice to be far too simplistic. In future projects I would still be as rigorous as possible in designing and conducting the research, but I suspect I would be more careful before automatically attributing the same motivations and investments regarding participation to disabled and non-disabled people alike. I know too, that as a result of working through this process I have gained insights into aspects of non-disabled people's experience to which I would not otherwise have had access. As a result,

I now firmly believe that more disabled researchers should conduct research projects with non-disabled people, as a way of exploring and seeking to understand their world-view, and of uncovering similarities and differences in our approaches both to research and to life in general. Such studies would provide a valuable, indeed essential, addition to the existing body of work on pathways to inclusion.

The importance of data triangulation in uncovering constructions of disability

In much of this chapter to date I have concentrated on discussing the formal interview situations at Greenways from which some of the research findings were derived. However, interviewing was not the only research method I used. As I have already mentioned, before the fieldwork began concerns had been raised as to whether I, as a disabled person, would be able to ask non-disabled people about their constructions of disability and expect honest answers in return. In response to this objection, I drew on Cohen and Manion's view (1994: 234) that the more different the techniques a researcher uses, the more confident s/he can be that the results are not accidental. In this project, I therefore used triangulation between observation, participation, document analysis and what people said at interview to check the accuracy of my initial interpretations before drawing any major conclusions. Sometimes I would watch one activity class over several weeks to check for similarities and differences, both in what happened and in how people related to each other, while interviews provided particularly useful opportunities to obtain respondent validation (or otherwise) of what I had previously observed (Hammersley and Atkinson, 1983: 195–8). Within the interviews themselves I then used a further form of triangulation in that I always asked people about their experiences of working with people from a range of minority groups, not just with disabled people. In so doing I hoped to explore the general effectiveness or otherwise of the Centre's equal opportunities policies, and to see whether positive or negative attitudes displayed towards any one minority group were generalized to others. Some of the results of this particular exercise are discussed in Chapter 9. However, achieving full triangulation in this way was not always possible. Some staff left the organization before they could be formally interviewed, while one or two others behaved towards me in such a hostile or negative manner that I decided it would be asking too much of myself to interview them one to one. Sometimes, though, interviews were not needed to confirm either discriminatory or inclusive practice.

The day of my gym induction session showed up unexpected barriers to inclusion. When I first met the fitness instructor who was to conduct the induction he appeared on the surface to be quite upbeat and friendly, though he clearly had a set spiel to get through, from which he wasn't going to be distracted by any attempts at general conversation. I later learned that usually in the New Year a lot of people join gyms as a way of getting fit after their Christmas excesses, but that they often give up again within weeks. It might well have been, then, that he didn't see much point in wasting a lot of time on social niceties until he was convinced I was going to be a serious long-term customer; and certainly I was not altogether sure, especially at the start, that he was actually listening to what I was saying during our conversation. For example, he asked me if I could fill in a card giving my name and address, so I replied by saying it would be easier if he did it. He said that was fine, and then thirty seconds later he handed me the blank card to fill in. I was so unnerved by this gulf between what he'd said and what he'd done that I didn't do anything to put the situation right. It now became clear that either he had made no attempt to understand me first time round, or that he was so scared at being with me that he simply could not take in anything I was saying. It felt easiest to go along with what he wanted, so I started filling in the form. Very quickly, however, he took it back when he realized he couldn't read it, even though I'd only got as far as writing 'Claire'. He scored my writing through deeply, and then took down the details at my dictation. I didn't like this – it seemed to rub in how far my writing falls short of the mark that he needed to eradicate it, so that it did not sully his clean card.

Next he gave me an information pack, and underlined the busy times 'so you can avoid them'. By this time, though, I wasn't too sure if this was really for my benefit, or whether it was designed to avoid too many other people having to train alongside me. After that he showed me a health form. Glancing cursorily at it, I noted that it appeared to mainly deal with things like chest pain which were not factors usually related to my particular impairment. Because of this, I offered to fill it in there and then, but instead he told me to take it away and 'get someone to go through it with you'. He actually used this phrase four times during the hour's induction session. I felt very undermined by this, as it clearly implied that either: (a) I wouldn't understand the questions; or (b) might not fill the form in properly. I really wasn't sure where this came from, since on the surface both his manner and his approach to trying to meet my needs were otherwise fairly good, and definitely seemed to improve in the course of the session, as he relaxed and began to understand my speech as a matter of routine. At this point I decided I was prepared to chalk his initial inappropriate behaviour down to lack of experience, and so I didn't dwell on his comments afterwards.

What changed my mind, and made me realize that he had after all been actively discriminating against me, was that a week later I happened upon him running through an induction session with some apparently visibly non-disabled people. By way of making a comparison with my own experience, I decided to see what happened, so I hung round at the next table making notes while he again went through his introductory spiel.

This time I noticed that he was rushing through it all very quickly, as if he couldn't wait to get the formalities out of the way so he could move on to demonstrating the equipment – which I guess is probably how the inductees felt too. What I found interesting, though, was that he didn't tell them to take the health forms home and get someone to go through them, as he had done with me, but just told them to fill them in there and then, and he would witness them. I realized from this that in my case he hadn't wanted to take responsibility for allowing me to use the equipment, and had instead wanted to invoke the added authority of some supposed third party who knew me to confirm it was OK for me to participate. It was also interesting that he hadn't felt he could be honest with me about his concerns. So although on the surface I had the same access to the gym facilities as everyone else, the conditions for my acceptance there were different. I guess that's one of the differences between superficial integration and real inclusion.

Sometimes, however, triangulation threw up positive changes in people's behaviour towards me over time, as they became more used to me being around. For example, during one early site visit I went to the café, where I was served by someone I hadn't met before. Immediately I picked up disapproval of me, in the way she said 'yes, James *said* you could have the staff discount' after I'd said I was entitled to it. It was as if she thought this was an unnecessary indulgence on his part. Certainly her manner made me instantly decide not to give her my purse so she could get the money out herself, which is what I usually do in shops, because I did not feel that she had yet earned that level of trust from me. Nor did she ask me where I wanted to sit, so I let her put my drink where she wanted – at the table nearest the till, as it happened. This was actually quite inconvenient for me, as it was furthest away from where the action was in the pool that I was hoping to observe, but somehow her manner made me decide not to comment. Had I been an ordinary paying customer I would then have made sure that I never used the café again when she was on duty, as this is the sort of small-scale hassle I do not need. However, as a researcher there were some situations where I felt I had to put my own feelings on hold in pursuit of collecting data, so a couple of weeks later I tried again. I did not really hold out much hope of a change, especially since this was a Sunday morning, the café was full and the staff were really busy. However, this time she was completely different. She came out from behind the counter, poured my drink, took my money, told her colleague on the till that I was entitled to the staff discount, put my change away for me, asked me if I wanted a straw, and then asked where I wanted to sit. This was a startling contrast to her previous 'let's get rid of this person as soon as possible' approach. Later I glanced across and caught her eye, and she smiled back. I was completely amazed, and delighted, at this positive transformation. In the absence of other evidence, it seemed likely that over time she had simply got used to seeing me around the place, so she was no longer frightened of me, and now felt confident of her own ability to treat me as an ordinary customer. Alternatively, it may have been the case that she had discussed our previous encounter with colleagues, and had taken their advice on how to behave around me in future. More generally, the experience was also one of several which helped confound my initial expectation that staff would be less prepared to provide a personalized service when they were busy. Throughout the fieldwork I experienced the same levels of service during both busy and slack times. Although this is only as it should be, it was nice to have my initial pessimism overturned.

An unexpected additional form of triangulation available to me as a disabled person derived from my decision to use a support worker during the research. This came about mainly because I find writing by hand difficult, and so I needed someone who could take notes for me in situations where the use of a tape recorder would have been inappropriate or technically impossible. In the pool area, for example, there was so much background noise that using a tape recorder just would not have worked, and when observing some of the group activities any recording of my observations would have been audible to the participants. In these situations, using a support worker seemed the best alternative, so Jill joined me towards the end of my second month at Greenways, and worked with me for around six weeks. Right from the start, however, I discovered that her presence had an effect on my own interactions with the staff. By this time I felt that I was on casual conversation terms with most people, and that they were becoming fairly comfortable with me being around the place. However, I was shocked to find that as soon as they had a choice between talking to me and talking to her, a non-disabled stranger, several of them immediately ignored me and spoke to her instead, even though I had made it clear before her arrival that I was her employer and therefore nominally 'in charge'. Their actions struck me as a blatant example of exclusion.

After this had happened a few times Jill and I talked about it, and as a result decided that in future she would only accompany me on half my site visits, as I could not risk all my previous work on building fieldwork relationships being wiped out due to people's preference for talking to her rather than me. This was also the main reason why we only worked together for six weeks in all. Once the general observation stage was over, and I had started using the tape recorder more routinely, I was able to continue the fieldwork alone. However, what threw the staff's reactions into even sharper relief was the positive and inclusive way in which disabled people at Greenways responded to Jill's presence. None of them ignored her and spoke only to me, and they would often ask after her on days when I was working by myself. Most simply took it for granted that I should be using a support worker, and sometimes it felt like I became seen as more trustworthy than before because I was using the same sort of support tools as they themselves were. Members of one group in particular took her under their wing and did all they could to make her feel at home, including encouraging me to take part in some of their activities so that she would be allowed to join in as well. From what she's told me I know that she felt privileged to be shown such care and concern.

Challenging oppression alongside non-disabled people

In terms of the work itself, Jill proved to be highly competent, and her general awareness of disability issues also made her a valuable ally and sounding board for some of my reflections on why people were acting in particular ways. I also found that sometimes her interpretations of people's behaviour were far less generous than my own. I know that in the interests of minimizing my identity bias I tended to play down or find alternative explanations for some instances of oppression, but she had no such qualms. It made me realize how much – both as a researcher and as a disabled person – I had been conditioned not to rock the boat too much, in case future access to fieldwork settings was denied. Strictly speaking, of course, it might be argued that I should not have discussed the research with her, because in a technical sense she was not a researcher herself. However, there was a confidentiality clause written into her contract, and she was present at a number of important encounters. In fact, on one occasion when I was becoming uneasy about the treatment of a group of disabled people, it was having my suspicions confirmed by her independent account that finally swung the balance and made me decide to take action. What followed in that situation is discussed more fully in Chapter 13.

Several times, having immediate access to her 'take' on what we were seeing also proved incredibly useful when people used dialect expressions in describing disabled people. As an outsider to the area, I didn't always understand what these phrases meant or what they additionally implied, and more than once Jill's translations were needed to reveal people's real discomfort at being with disabled people. Equally, however, there were times when my own access to insider codes left her at a loss. One time a disabled woman whom I'd got to know came over for a chat, and said she'd just been in the gym, so I said I used it too, and had quite enjoyed it. She continued with 'yes, if you tell people straight up, then they're usually all right, but if you try to bluff your way through . . .' at which point I said 'yes, I agree'. And that was all we said. When she'd gone I turned to Jill and said 'did you get that?' and she said 'get what?'. So then we talked about it, and about why the conversation was important (i.e. that if you explain your impairment needs upfront then people are usually quite suppor-tive, but if you don't then you can end up in sticky situations). Having to unpeel and explain that short exchange showed me how much of it had in fact been mediated by unspoken shared cultural knowledge to which Jill was not privy, so it had made no real sense to her. This in turn made me realize that if we do need to develop a common language with which to discuss disability issues, then it's not only non-disabled people who will have to look again at their existing practice.

Working with Jill was the first time that I had used a support worker during fieldwork. I found it a largely positive experience, and one which made me reflect more regularly and in greater depth on some of the assumptions about the research that I had previously taken for granted. Often in working with her I found that I had to be more explicit about my decision-making processes than would have been the case had I been working alone, in order that she understood exactly what I expected of her in supporting the fieldwork. I am sure that this in turn further increased my own reflexivity both in developing appropriate ways of conducting the fieldwork, and in carrying out the subsequent data analysis. However, employing someone in this capacity also had undoubted implications for the management of the project, in terms of needing to allow additional time for recruitment, confirming funding for the post, and meeting the employee's training and support needs, which would not affect a researcher who was able to work entirely independently. As Zarb (1997) has previously pointed out, such factors must always be borne in mind when research projects likely to involve disabled researchers are first being planned, so that additional time and resources are included to meet potential support and training needs. Otherwise some disabled people will continue to be prevented from playing a full part in the research community.

The generally negative effect that Jill's presence had on my interactions with other non-disabled people at Greenways also led me to begin to question the efficacy of the normalization/SRV premise that encouraging disabled people to mix with non-disabled people may represent their best hope of social acceptance (Wolfensberger, 1992). I will explore other aspects of this premise in later chapters that deal more particularly with the exclusionary experiences of people with learning difficulties at Greenways. For now I simply want to make the point that even for me, as a skilled professional researcher apparently already engaged in a range of socially valued roles alongside non-disabled people, this was not always enough to guarantee my full inclusion. As I have shown, the mere presence of a non-disabled support worker was enough to make the non-disabled research participants feel that they no longer had to make the effort to engage with me direct, and that they could instead fall back on the easier option of communicating with her as a fellow non-disabled person. This finding suggests that simply bringing disabled and non-disabled people together, sometimes even using the mediation of a support worker to facilitate the interaction (Race, 1999), is not in itself enough to achieve real inclusion. There is always the risk that while such encounters continue to be based on the deeply ingrained normative assumption that non-disabled people represent what is normal and safe, disabled people will continue to be excluded.

Some conclusions

Overall as a result of my experiences of being a researcher at Greenways I would say that, contrary to initial concerns, it is possible for disabled people to uncover aspects of non-disabled people's construction of disability. Certainly, at one level the relationship of trust which I built up over time with the staff at Greenways appeared to enable them to be relatively honest in what they told me. A number named their own fear, embarrassment and uncertainty around disabled customers as being barriers to equal service provision. Few made overtly politically correct statements, and where they did it was usually possible to evaluate what they said against how I had previously seen them act. Some of what I was told did not match up with what I had seen, and most times I preferred to rely on my own instinct and prior experience of oppression in making sense of these competing accounts.

Overall, then, I can argue that I did uncover at least some 'real' constructions of disability. And yet, the triangulation safeguard I had introduced into the interview phase of asking people their views about other minority groups also made me realize some of the limitations of my research. Specifically, what other white people told me honestly of their views on black and Asian people using the Centre (discussed in Chapter 9) suggests that, similarly, if I had been a non-disabled person some of them might also have been more candid in some aspects of what they told me about impairment and disability. For the future, then, on any similar projects I would like to try working with a non-disabled researcher, to see if this approach allowed a wider range of data to be uncovered. Having said that, the experience in this setting of having people prefer to talk to my non-disabled support worker rather than to me has also made me realize the need to build appropriate safeguards into any such collaborative project, to minimize the risk of the same thing happening again. Simple ways of achieving this might be for each of us to visit the setting at separate times or on different days, or by using a combination of individual and joint visits to compare people's reactions. Even given the limitations of the present research, however, it has undoubtedly given me a range of insights into non-disabled thinking which I could not otherwise have imagined.

Some of the scenes I observed or was part of at Greenways were personally oppressive to me, a situation which I found increasingly hard to accept over time as I became more familiar with staff and customers in the setting, and thus came to expect routinely inclusive treatment. Given such stresses, it was essential throughout to have access to a support network within the wider research community, so that I didn't go under. Developing a support network is a valuable resource for any research project which is personally involving, and one which I would recommend to other researchers. Another strategy I used was to make firm decisions about when not to continue, and whom not to interview, where going into such a situation was most likely only to lead to more personal oppression. I adopted this self-protection strategy because I felt that some data was just not worth having if the personal cost was too high. Again, I suspect that working with a non-disabled person would have been useful in some of those situations, where it would have been of value to the project to have interviewed someone who was exhibiting all the signs of oppressive behaviour, but where I felt it would be asking too much of myself to do so. Thus in much the same way as male researchers could support feminist research by working in male environments which are too inaccessible or dangerous for women researchers to enter (Griffin and Weatherell, 1992: 148), so I believe non-disabled researchers could support disability research by interviewing the worst of the oppressors.

In the next chapter I turn to a discussion of how my identity as a consultant enabled me both to explore the extent to which the organizational structure and policies of the leisure centre facilitated the creation of inclusive recreation opportunities there, and to evaluate how much of an effect such structures had on the behaviour of individual members of staff.

Chapter 5

Being a consultant

The impact of my professional background on the research

As mentioned in the Introduction, my background as a countryside recreation professional was a major factor in my decision to study constructions of disability within the leisure industry. For this research project I knew I wanted to work in an environment where I already understood a range of the issues, problems and approaches, so that I would have a greater chance of being able to place what I was seeing within the wider context of developments within that field. However, I was not sure that going back specifically to countryside recreation would be wise, since it is an area in which I have been too immersed, and to which I would bring too many preconceptions and prejudices. Hence my decision to take a sideways step to work at a leisure centre. I knew that there would be some issues and approaches that such a venue would have in common with countryside sites, but that equally there would be some new factors to discover, and different connections to be made. I found this prospect exciting, and could see in it potential benefits for my further professional development.

At the start of my access negotiations with Greenways, however, I took the decision to play down my previous professional experience, since I did not want to raise expectations with the staff that my main role at the site would be to sort out all their access problems for them. For this project my main focus had to be on uncovering constructions of disability, and I could not risk being sidetracked from that aim into becoming an unpaid access officer. That said, there were some aspects of my previous working practice which I knew I wanted to use here. In particular, I had been used to developing projects based on the concept of praxis, bringing together disabled and non-disabled people to develop workable solutions to existing access problems. In such cases, theory and practice had developed from each other in a mutual cyclical relationship (Carr and Kemmis, 1986: 34). This is at heart a profoundly optimistic way of working, based on a belief that by bringing practitioners and service users together and utilizing all their skills and knowledge, improved policy and practice can be achieved. It would have been easy to have fallen back on this method of cooperative working at Greenways, and to have developed a project based wholly on action research principles. I know that this strategy works, and I suspect that we would have achieved more access improvements at the site, and more quickly, had I used this as my only methodological approach. However, I also knew from previous professional experience that this sort of collaboration tends to appeal most to those staff who are already generally in favour of the concept of inclusion, and who actively want to find ways of improving their practice. At Greenways, had I chosen only to work with people like that, I would have missed out on the possibility of also uncovering the perspectives of those to whom the idea of inclusion is less attractive. Hence, for this project, deciding to try to work with all the staff enabled me to study people with a wider range of views. This was important because, at the end of the day, inclusion will only succeed if the reluctant as well as the committed can be persuaded of its merits and possibilities.

Problems and opportunities of being seen as a consultant

At the start of the fieldwork I experienced some qualms about 'contaminating' my researcher identity with that of the consultant. Apart from my concerns about coming to be seen solely as an access officer, I was also worried that staff awareness of my professional expertise might make them more wary about my motives, and suspicious that I was only there to find fault with their performance. This was a particular concern because observation soon showed that the organization's transition from the public to the private sector, and the resulting increased pressure to generate income, was making many of the staff nervous. Although some did appear to revel in the resultant new opportunities to develop their skills and to take on more responsibility, others were clearly fearful for their job security, and a number did actually leave the organization during the course of the fieldwork. In retrospect, discovering all this made me regret originally telling the staff that I was there to look at community use of the Centre, as I am sure that – despite my assurances to the contrary – some of them initially saw this as a cover for a time and motion study designed to check up on their performance. Certainly it helps to explain some staff reactions to me during my first site visit, when I quickly became aware that they were 'checking me out' as they went by, with some smiling half self-consciously as they passed, while others studiously ignored my presence. To begin with that day I sat by the pool making a few notes, but after a while I realized that there was an increased tension in the air, and looking up I saw apprehension in people's faces as they focused on my notebook. Clearly it was time for me to move on.

As a result of this experience, over the first few weeks in particular I was careful not to spend too much time in any one place, so that people would feel less threatened by me. I also had a lot of informal chats with a range of members of staff, which were designed to reduce their fear of my difference. Although I did not feel comfortable about adopting an approach based on the assumption that it was me who was different from them, rather than that we were different from each other, I knew that to start with this was probably how they would see the situation. As a result, I was prepared to play along with such perceptions until such time as we got to know each other better. Some of the ways in which we did later start to question binary assumptions around sameness and difference are discussed in subsequent chapters. For now, though, I must admit that colluding with mainstream assumptions about my own difference did have the desired effect of enabling people to decide that as a disabled person I did not pose a threat to their own positions of relative power, and that as such they could relax and tell me more about themselves.

It was at this stage that I began to discover the full extent of their concerns about job security during this time of organizational change. This was something which I could identify with, having been through a similar experience in my own career. The unexpected opportunity which this commonality presented to share our thoughts and feelings on this issue, and for me to be able to tell them some of the approaches to managing the situation which had seen me through my own experience of organizational change, was an important factor in breaking down the initial barriers between us. On the downside, though, I know that it also led in this respect to an over-identification on my part with the staff's experience which was in turn instrumental in my consultant identity being as important as it was to the research. More positively, I could also say that this was a situation in which I had the contacts, knowledge, tools and power to do something to improve matters, whereas many of the staff did not. Put simply, in this aspect of their identity they were disabled here, not me. Once I realized this, I decided that taking on an advocacy role, rather than simply reporting their lack of empowerment, was an appropriate response. This eventually led me, at the end of the fieldwork, to produce a consultancy report for the management which included the anonymized reporting of some widespread staff concerns about Greenways policy and practice. More generally, although it was at odds with my belief that in general disabled people should not be expected to conduct advisory work for free, I also accepted the fact that I was not paid for any of the consultancy work I carried out there, since in this case it was part of the payback for being granted free access to the site and use of the facilities to conduct the research.

As the fieldwork progressed and I demonstrated increasing competence in the setting, I actually found that some of the Centre managers became less helpful towards me than they had been to begin with. I can only assume that this was because once they realized I had a fairly wide range of practical skills, which I was indeed using to assess policy and practice at the site, they could no longer simply dismiss me as a relatively powerless outsider/ researcher. Coming to be seen as a threat in this way caused me some problems, especially in relation to my requests for statistical information about the site. Inevitably, such requests either took at least two months to be met, or somehow just didn't happen at all. I also noticed that during my familiarization visits I was not shown where either the managers' offices or the staff room were, and picked up the message from this that as an outsider/consultant these areas were closed to me. I did not make any attempt to access these rooms independently, as I thought people would see it as snooping, and that I might be asked to leave the site as a result. Some two months later James did say I could use the staff room, and – if he was with me – the offices. However, by now it would have felt too artificial to have suddenly started doing so, and I only actually went into the staff room once during the whole seven months. I am aware that as a result of this decision there were some staff whom I never met, or whose roles even now I cannot identify, but my only real option was to accept this as a limitation of the research. Later on in the project, though, I did, with his permission, use James' room independently for meetings on a few occasions. I know that this action confirmed some people's assumptions that I was working for him. By that stage, though, it mattered far less than it would have done at the beginning, when I had felt it necessary to do all I could to distance myself from him to avoid just such assumptions being made. A key reason for my later more relaxed approach was that by then I felt I had established myself within the setting in my own right, a transition which came about largely as a result of my interventions in support of staff initiatives to improve access.

This decision may seem contradictory in the light of my earlier statement that I did not want to become Greenways' unpaid access officer. However, this determination coexisted with my political desire to work with the staff to make at least some changes to policy and practice. Actually I would have found it almost impossible to have carried out my research without taking account of the prevailing access barriers and doing something to remove them, an approach which I could justify by the agreement made with Greenways at the start of the research that my findings would be used by them to improve existing policy and practice. Hence when, in my first month on site, the marketing officer mentioned that he was about to produce a new series of corporate publicity leaflets, I felt it was appropriate to give him a set of guidelines on accessible design, covering issues such as print size, language and colour contrast, so that the new leaflets were more user-friendly than the old ones had been. Similarly, on only my third site visit I was asked to undertake a comprehensive audit of the accessible toilets. As a result of such interventions, by the mid-point of my fieldwork

I had produced a thirty-point action plan of repair work and recommended access improvements, which I was told would be implemented once the Centre refurbishment took place. Some unexpected outcomes of my taking on this additional role are discussed in Chapters 6 and 13. For now, I want to concentrate on the effect which such interventions had on my relationships with the staff. Specifically, it felt like because they could see that I was putting my consultancy skills at their disposal in a supportive way, and not simply trying to find fault with their performance, I now became seen as more trustworthy. As time went on, people would often stop by for a chat, to ask how the research was going and to give me more information which they felt would be useful to me.

Links and gaps between policy and practice at Greenways

As the research progressed, it became evident that there were a number of structural barriers to disabled people's inclusion at Greenways. The most obvious example of this lay in the provision of differential physical access to some of the activity areas. For example, for mainstream customers, access to the sports hall was via the changing rooms. However, there was a heavy-duty steel barrier in front of the changing rooms, which appeared to bar the route to wheelchair users. In actual fact this was not the case, since the central part of the barrier could easily be pushed open. However, it appeared that nobody had explained to the members or staff of the segregated disability groups who used the Centre that this was the case, so instead they routinely accessed the sports hall via fire doors and a separate corridor which were clearly marked 'No Entry' to members of the public. Indeed, Greenways staff actively encouraged this practice by propping the fire doors open for them. As a result, the group members gained functional access to the sports hall, but only through special segregated access provision which was both unnecessary and which further served to reinforce notions that disabled people were different and needed to be separated off from other users. Shortly after I finished my fieldwork, the steel barrier in front of the changing rooms was in fact removed, as an initial step towards improving access. It is also intended that the whole of the changing areas will be made accessible once the planned Centre refurbishment takes place. However, unless Centre staff have also stopped opening the fire doors for the groups, and started encouraging them to go through the changing rooms instead, this will have been a purely cosmetic exercise, and differential access to the facilities will remain the norm.

During the formal interview stage of the fieldwork I wanted to find out how aware the Centre staff were of disabling barriers at the site, and so I asked each interviewee what they thought were the main problems that might put disabled people off using the facility. Although some of them started off by saying that they thought the existing access provision was good, they then always asked me for my opinion, and seemed to be prepared to learn from my experience of aspects of provision which made the Centre difficult to use. Others showed pre-existing high levels of awareness of disabling barriers. Problems mentioned included the high prices charged for entry, the lack both of general publicity information about the Centre's facilities and of targeted information provision aimed specifically at disabled people, a general lack of accessible public transport in the town, and the abuse by non-disabled drivers of car parking spaces reserved for disabled people at the site. As discussed in Chapter 10, one person suggested that Greenhills should offer more segregated disabled-only sessions as a means of building people's confidence prior to their participation in mainstream activities, while others highlighted the need to reassure potential customers with impairments that Centre staff were fully trained and would be able to meet their requirements. The idea of taster days was also raised as a way of enabling disabled people to visit the site to meet the staff, discuss any specific impairment-related sporting needs, and to try out some of the activities on offer.

Often the staff making these suggestions qualified them by saying that such initiatives were unlikely to be implemented in the current economic climate. However, as individuals many of them were clearly committed to both the principle and the practice of inclusion. Their responses also revealed an awareness of structural disabling barriers, including some, like the Centre's pricing policy mentioned above, which confirmed that othering of disabled people with low incomes on economic grounds did take place at the site. Further, the data also highlighted the interrelationship between the Centre and the wider environment, through the negative effect that a lack of targeted advertising within the wider community and an inaccessible public transport system were having on take-up of Centre facilities by disabled people. The advertising issue was one on which the Centre could take action, but developing an accessible transport system would rely on decision-making elsewhere. It may therefore be argued that individual projects to provide accessible venues will only become truly effective when the wider infrastructure of society is made equally accessible.

Another of the measures I used to assess the extent of inclusive practice at Greenways was the completion of a document analysis of selected organizational policies, as a means of uncovering links and gaps between policy and practice. In doing so, I was surprised to discover that actually Greenways had few written policies, other than those to do with personnel issues, and that they had no formal written recreation or visitor management strategies. Instead, I was told that most activities at the Centre were undertaken with the twin aims of income generation and debt reduction. In practice I discovered that this imperative had led to increasing competition between the various departments, as each sought to increase customer take-up of their own particular activities, sometimes with little regard for any negative knock-on effect this might have on other areas of the facility. This approach also led on occasion to mixed messages being given to customers. For example, one manager told me that disabled people could borrow flotation aids and mobility equipment in order to use the pool. This seemed a positive and proactive approach towards achieving inclusion, and was potentially a good marketing tool which might attract disabled people to the facility who could not afford to purchase such equipment for themselves. It also appeared to constitute a 'reasonable adjustment' in terms of Part III of the Disability Discrimination Act (1995), which stipulates that disabled people should have equal access to goods and services. However, when I asked another manager about this extra provision, I was told that only those disabled people who visited in formal groups could borrow such equipment, thus excluding anyone who visited as an individual. One of the recommendations of my final consultancy report was that such conflicts in policy and practice could be avoided in the future if agreed written guidelines on matters such as equipment loans and other aspects of service provision were produced and circulated to all staff, and incorporated in practical ways into their own performance targets, to generate a more cohesive organization-wide approach.

Document analysis of selected personnel policies uncovered similar anomalies. In some, for example, disabled people were described as valued employees and customers against whom discrimination would not be tolerated. In others, however, implicit negative value judgements were apparent. For example, in one it was stated that staff were eligible for an annual unpaid dependency leave allowance, which could be extended in 'special circumstances', including 'when the dependent is physically or mentally handicapped'. This policy can be criticized both for its use of inappropriate descriptive terminology, and for its assumption that disabled people will be sick and need care more often than non-disabled people. This assumption might in turn make staff unconsciously reluctant to consider recruiting new members of staff who have impairments, in the mistaken belief that such staff would inevitably take a lot of sick leave. More positively, however, another policy stated that where an existing employee acquired an impairment which affected the range of duties which s/he was able to perform, then a range of specific remedial options must be explored, with the emphasis being on retaining the employee within the organization wherever possible. As a result of this document analysis, a number of issues are now being addressed by the organization at a corporate level to resolve existing anomalies in its personnel policies as they relate to disabled people and other minority groups.

Another barrier uncovered during the research was the relative lack of a staff training policy. Training to meet essential health and safety requirements was provided, but other forms of staff development were not routinely offered. Although many staff did act in a proactive way to deal with unexpected issues, and some even appeared to positively relish being 'thrown in at the deep end', from my observation others were clearly uneasy about dealing with disabled people, and most reported a desire for more training so that they could further improve their service delivery. In fact, two of the formal interviews I held with staff turned into impromptu disability equality training sessions, as they sought my advice on ways of making their own working practice more inclusive. On the other hand, some staff clearly already had well-developed skills in delivering equal services to people with and without impairments. However, another consequence of the interdepartmental rivalry was the compartmentalization of skills and knowledge, so that such experience was not routinely shared across the organization. More positively, however, although training provision was not improved while this research was underway, anecdotal evidence received since then suggests that more courses are now being made available to staff.

Exclusionary practice among external contractors

During the research it became apparent that not all of the external contractors who ran sessions at Greenways adopted the same generally inclusive approach to service provision as did Centre staff. Since all of the formal disabled-only sessions at the Centre were run by external contractors (often local Council disability support services staff), this meant that on occasion I witnessed exclusionary treatment of disabled people which I know would not have been tolerated had it been delivered by Greenways staff. Some examples and possible explanations for this discrimination are discussed in Chapter 11. The specific point I want to make here is that the organization's anti-discrimination policy appeared to have a positive effect on the behaviour of Greenways' own staff, but not always on that of the contractors. This is perhaps not surprising, since such contractors were in effect customers of the Centre, who paid a fee to use the facilities for teaching sessions with their groups. Even so, the organization's anti-discrimination policy was on public display in a number of places around the Centre, so nobody using the facility, whether staff or customers, could use the excuse that they did not know what such policies were.

The finding that Greenways staff behaved inclusively most of the time might be used as a strong argument in favour of organizational anti-discrimination policies, which it is. Yet at the same time a note of caution must be added, in that policies can only work if they are fully implemented. At the start of this research, it seemed that little was being done by the management at Greenways to address the exclusionary behaviour of contractors at the site. It appeared either that Centre staff were unaware of the inappropriate behaviour of these contractors, or that they felt unable to challenge the ways in which other professionals went about their business.

I found this apparent lack of action confusing and contradictory, and at odds with the Centre's own policies. In retrospect, however, I now realize that such contradictions are probably fairly commonplace, and are an indication of the extent to which settings do not exist in isolation, but are affected by wider events, behaviours and attitudes. Thus some of the external support services staff were able to import into this setting standards of behaviour around disabled people which must have been tolerated in other settings, but which were at odds with the more inclusive ethos of Greenways, simply because their status as 'disability professionals' and holders of exclusive knowledge about working with disabled people made them appear beyond reproach.

The exclusionary behaviour of some disability professionals further reinforced the research finding that no one setting can be studied in isolation. This is supported by evidence from other research, such as Gillborn and Youdell's study (2000: 220) of inequality of educational opportunity in two London schools, in which they concluded that 'processes at both the macro *and* micro levels are implicated in the current iniquitous status quo'. Thus at Greenways, processes at the macro level, including the exclusionary approaches towards disabled people brought into the setting by some disability contractors, had an undoubted negative impact on the quality of leisure services offered at micro level to those customers. That such differential behaviour existed between Greenways staff and external contractors also suggests the primacy of economic factors in influencing constructions of disability. Staff working for and paid a regular salary by Greenways usually acted in an inclusive way, whereas external contractors who simply used the Centre as a temporary working space did not always do so. Nor could Centre customers automatically be expected to know whether they were being taught by Greenways staff or by contractors. Hence it is likely that those who did experience discrimination at the hands of trainers, coaches and support staff will have assumed that those staff simply mirrored Greenways' general approach. This is extremely unfortunate, since overall I, as an individual customer who usually took part in Centre-run activities, found the setting to be one of the most relaxed and inclusive places I have ever worked in. However, from my observations it seemed clear both that disabled people who visited Greenways as part of contractor-run groups were not always treated in respectful and inclusive ways, and that in the absence of any evidence to the contrary, they will have assumed that such treatment was routine for customers of the Centre.

Some conclusions

Although I was initially reticent about 'contaminating' my identity as a researcher with that of a consultant, it was undoubtedly the case that being able to draw on both aspects of my experience in collecting data for the project added an extra dimension to my findings. Arguably, it was my consultancy skills which allowed me the greatest access to policy information (Schein, 1987), since this was an area of reportedly little in-house staff knowledge, and hence one where they could see direct benefits to the organization from my input. Some of this access might have been difficult to obtain had I stuck to my original ethnographic intention of simply reporting what was happening there at present. In some ways they already knew that – what they were looking for were ideas on what they could do about it. Equally, though, had my involvement at the site been solely with management and policy issues I would not have been able to investigate how things worked at grassroots level. I would therefore argue that being able to address approaches to inclusion from both angles was crucial to uncovering a broader picture of what was happening there (ibid., 1987). After the fieldwork was over I was told that my input had led to changes in approach not just at Greenways, but also at other venues now managed by the same organization. At a personal level I found this extremely satisfying, and it did seem to vindicate my decision to use a combination of approaches in conducting this research.

In addition, I found that being able to study both policy and practice at once unsettled some of my initial assumptions and confirmed others. The differential practice of Greenways staff and some of the external contractors justified my decision to look at the effects of organizational policy on individual behaviour, but at the same time made me question the effectiveness of such policies. It may well be, of course, that in private or in other public settings some Greenways staff exhibited similarly overt discriminatory behaviour and beliefs towards disabled people to that shown by some of the contractors. However, the point was that in this particular setting they knew that such behaviour would not be tolerated. That the organization's equalities policy did seem to have a positive effect on employees' behaviour lends empirical support to the materialist social model argument that structural change, including the implementation of such anti-discrimination policies, is a necessary prerequisite to achieving inclusion. However, it did not deal with the problem of ongoing discrimination by some of the contractors. At a practical level, one way of ensuring future compliance on their part would be for their teaching sessions to be monitored and assessed against the Centre's equal opportunities policy, and then for the Centre to require any identified shortfalls to be addressed, or else permission to use the facilities would be withdrawn. In relation to some of the sessions run for disabled people, I also believe it would have been preferable for Greenways staff to have taken over the running of these groups, so that the same level of service would be offered to those group members as was routinely provided for independent Centre users. As things stood, the biggest structural barrier to inclusion appeared to be the role of disability professionals in running the disability groups. Their approach perpetuated negative images of disabled people as dependent service users rather than as economically valued customers, and as such perpetuated their exclusion. In suggesting that Centre staff should take over, I remain mindful of St Claire's finding (1986) that increased individual disabled/non-disabled interactions might simply lead to those non-disabled people being ascribed disabled people's devalued social status rather than, as intended, increasing disabled people's opportunities for social inclusion. However, at Greenways I believe that any such tendency would be more than outweighed by the strength of the economic imperative to provide a high level of service to customers, in case they otherwise decided to take their business elsewhere. Thus structural economic factors such as the need to generate more income from customers have the potential to influence directly positive attitude changes towards disabled people, as Barnes (1991) has previously argued.

Overall, these findings seem to offer partial verification of my original epistemological assumption that an individual's constructions of disability do not exist in isolation, but are also affected by the environments in which they find themselves. However, the important rider must now be added that it may be the fact of the combination of the social environment which the individual inhabits, together with their economic position, which has the potential to improve disabling attitudes. Put simply, if depressingly, Greenways staff knew they had to behave inclusively towards all customers, or risk losing their jobs. External contractors under no such immediate economic pressure did not always follow suit. This confirmed that no one setting can be studied in isolation, but must instead be seen in terms of the interconnectedness between inclusionary and exclusionary factors at both macro and micro level. In turn, this finding further vindicates the social model approach to explaining the ways that disability is created by a combination of cultural, organizational and economic factors, rather than seeing the issue as being purely one of relationships between individuals (Priestley, 1998). Thus inclusion is unlikely to be achieved solely through changing the attitudes of individual non-disabled people, but will also require wider action to remove structural barriers.

The next chapter continues to address the issue of gaps and connections between policy and practice at Greenways, as expressed through some of the tensions which I experienced in trying to combine my ascribed member of staff status with a more detached researcher and activist role. I also discuss how people's perceptions of me as a member of staff affected our relationships, and seemed to influence what they chose to reveal to me of their constructions of disability.

Chapter 6

Being a member of staff

Potential conflicts in identity and role

One identity I did not expect to be attributed to me at Greenways was that of being a member of staff. Indeed, in many ways, being ascribed staff status was anathema to my desire to be seen as an 'outsider' researcher and consultant, and it was never a role in which I felt personally comfortable. And, as discussed in the previous chapter, my access to some staff-only areas at Greenways was limited throughout the research, so it would not be true to say that I was ever regarded as a full member of the team in the same way that the regular members of staff were. However, there is no doubt that a number of staff and customers did come to see me as part of the Greenways scene, and that in some situations their belief that I was working for the organization led them to tell me things which they probably would not have revealed had they regarded me as either an ordinary customer or a detached researcher.

In ethical terms, being seen as a member of staff raised some big issues for me. For example, at the start of the research James made it clear to me that I would be expected to behave as Greenways staff did in my dealings with customers at the site. At one level this was perfectly understandable, in that he needed to be sure I would not do anything to embarrass the Centre publicly, or to upset or endanger the customers. However, I did find it necessary to resist some of his other suggestions intended to make me part of the scene. In the beginning he wanted me to have my own clocking-on card like the real members of staff, in order to add to the impression that I was working for the Centre, but I had problems with this at two levels. First, it would have misled the real staff into thinking that I was a colleague. In turn this might have made them consistently relate to me differently, especially if they thought I was working under contract to James, who had a reputation for championing equal opportunities without fear or favour. Although as mentioned previously it became clear that over time most people did indeed assume that I was working for him, at the beginning I knew that I needed to ensure I had done all I could to minimize the chances of being pigeonholed or thrust into stereotyped roles in this way. Second, I was aware that there were no people with obvious impairments working at the Centre. While appreciating the site's generosity in giving me access, I was conscious that there might be publicity benefits for them in appearing to have a disabled person working for the organization, especially one who happened to spend a lot of time in high-profile public access areas. I knew, therefore, that I had to manage this situation carefully to avoid giving the impression that Greenways was an equal opportunities employer of disabled people, when this was not necessarily the case. Thus, for example, on the specific clocking-in issue a compromise was reached whereby on each visit I signed in and out using the 'External Contractors' book. This satisfied health and safety regulations about needing to know who was on site in case there was an emergency of some kind, whilst avoiding the implication that I was a member of the Centre staff. This arrangement had the additional practical advantage for the research that often the duty officer would be there while I was signing in and out, so I could find out about any interesting events taking place that day, and get immediate feedback or additional information on issues which had arisen during that site visit.

More generally, the need to avoid being personally compromised in the ways described above was an added reason for my early decision to take on an overt access advisory role. As a disabled person, I did not want my presence at Greenways to be read by staff or customers either as an assurance that the site was fully physically and programme accessible, when clearly it was not, or as an indication that Greenways was an equal opportunities employer, when I was not actually on the payroll. As a consultant, I knew I had the skills and knowledge to help the Centre make positive access changes. And, as a putative member of staff, I was aware that I came to be seen in some quarters as someone who could influence James' management approach where others did not feel they themselves could do so. However, in order to minimize the impression that I was working solely for him, I also made sure that I spoke to, and developed links with, as many of the other staff and managers at Greenways as possible. This was in part because, as stated in the previous chapter, I believe that wholesale progress towards inclusion will only be achieved if everyone has a commitment to it, and not just a few people with expert knowledge. Also, of course, at the start of the fieldwork I could not take it for granted that James himself was a proactive force for change, or that he had the authority to persuade other people to adopt new working practices. Hence, in trying to make connections across the board at Greenways, I hoped to reinforce the idea that inclusion is an issue for everyone. As a result of this broad-based approach, I undoubtedly gained access to more information about organizational practices than I would have done had I relied on one or two particular staff contacts. Being able to use a range of skills to help improve access was also an important trade-off against the benefits for Greenways of having me there.

Some effects of my staff identity on people's constructions of disability

In a few cases I found that it was only once staff saw me as a productive member of the team that they were able to connect with me properly. This was especially true with one of the gym instructors. When I first started working out in the gym I found her manner rather offhand, an impression supported by unsolicited anecdotal evidence from some of the non-disabled customers. Their comments made me wary at first of attributing her unhelpful approach to a specific fear or dislike of me as a disabled person. However, subsequent interactions between us made me realize that at least part of her offhandedness with me did result from discomfort around my impairment. For example, in the early stages of the fieldwork I needed help getting on and off some of the pieces of equipment, and whilst other members of staff were always ready to oblige, I noticed that she had a tendency to vanish routinely at the critical moment. On the one occasion when I did pin her down and ask for her help, she visibly recoiled at the prospect of having to touch my foot in order to place it in the pedal strap of the exercise bike, and then quickly left the room once she'd done it, possibly for fear that I would ask her for further help. Actually her actions here had potentially serious health and safety implications, because at the end of my work-out I was left stranded on the bike, unable to get off it until another customer came to my aid. It appeared, then, that her fear of difference was so strong that it overrode any work-related responsibilities. In turn, this was the one occasion when I was tempted to name and shame a member of Greenways staff, because her actions had left me in such a vulnerable and potentially dangerous position. The reason I did not do so was purely research-related, in that the incident happened so early on in the fieldwork that I felt sure any complaint I made at that stage would destroy the relationships of trust which I was slowly building up with other members of staff, and might in fact make it impossible to carry on with the study.

However, the episode did have a practical knock-on effect for the progress of the fieldwork. It made me realize that, although I had the task as a researcher of investigating the nature of disabling practice at the Centre, I also had a duty of personal self-preservation. For some time afterwards I avoided using the gym when she was there, because I needed to be sure I could rely on the staff to help out if I got into difficulty. However, one day I bumped into her in the corridor while I was laden down with tape measure and clipboard, conducting an access audit. Seeing me in this 'official' role, she stopped and for the first time initiated a conversation with me. In my view, she only felt confident enough to do this because now she could classify me as a fellow member of staff (apparently) doing a job for James, whereas before she could only see me as a disabled person/customer. Although I cannot say that this event marked the start of a beautiful friendship, it did mark a breakthrough in that afterwards she felt able to speak to me from time to time about access issues, and also did less to avoid me when I was in the gym.

Gaining access to privileged information

It was in my staff role that I was eventually able to find out what lay behind the Centre's apparent harsh treatment, and eventual exclusion, of a customer with learning difficulties, actions which on the surface seemed to go against not just their equal opportunities policy but the generally inclusive feel of the place. Over a period of months I had often noticed this woman, Vicky, hanging around outside the building with her sports bag as if she was waiting for someone. I would smile and say hello, but she always ignored me. This was quite unusual, in that generally speaking Greenways was a friendly place, and most people would smile and exchange greetings in passing, even if they didn't know you by name. Then another time I saw her being escorted to where she wanted to go by a lifeguard who kept a firm grip on her arm so she couldn't get away, and who threatened to get James if she didn't 'behave'. Once I even heard her being asked to leave the Centre altogether, but without any apparent explanation being given. Clearly, then, she was well known to the staff, but I never saw her speak, and nobody ever explained what was going on, or why she was being excluded. Seeing these incidents in isolation, without benefit of an explanation, gave me the impression that the Centre was discriminating against her because of her impairment. Yet, knowing what I did by then of Centre policy and practice, this conclusion did not make sense.

Then one day as I was sitting in the upper lobby I noticed her heading my way. Two members of staff were also in the area, and when she saw them she stopped and began fiddling with her watchstrap, as if hoping that she would thereby render herself invisible. Straightaway it felt like something wasn't right. One of the staff turned round in his tracks and started off downstairs again, as if to get help. And then one of the managers arrived, and said – uncharacteristically sharply – 'Vicky, I want a word with you!'. She stopped by the lift, where they were too far away for me to be able to hear anything of what passed between them. However, in the time they were talking several other members of staff went by, and I was able to note down what they said – and they did all pass comment on the situation.

Lifeguard 1:   'hast tha been a bad girl again?' (Vicky looks in her twenties
to me).
Secretary: 'Have you been up to summat, Vicky?'
Lifeguard 2: (to the manager)   '. . . though it might have been nothing this
    time.'

I drew a number of conclusions from these comments. First, it appeared that
Vicky was well known to many of the staff by her first name (and sometimes
familiarity isn't generated for positive reasons). Second, she was being
treated by them like a naughty child (though I couldn't hear what the
manager was saying, so I don't know if she was doing this as well). Third,
she was assumed to be guilty of something – perhaps even before the facts
had been checked. Finally, I felt sure they would not have spoken to or
about her in such patronizing terms if she hadn't had learning difficulties.
Come to that, I had never previously heard Centre staff speak like that to
any other customers with learning difficulties. So, there must have been
something about this particular situation which was making them act in
such a publicly unprofessional way.

Later that day as I was signing out I casually asked the manager what
the story was, adding that I'd tried but failed to connect with Vicky
myself. I suppose in the way I phrased this I was lining myself up on 'her
side' as someone else who had trouble with this disabled person. This probably wasn't very ethical, but I did it because I wanted to see if she'd tell
me her side of the story, and I didn't think I'd get this if I took the moral
high ground. Somewhat to my surprise, she did then tell me her account.
Apparently Vicky had a history of carrying out acts of petty vandalism at
the Centre, and although meetings had been held with her, her parents and
her social worker to try to resolve the situation amicably, she had kept on
doing it. Recently she had been banned for a few weeks, but resumed her
old behaviour once readmitted. As a result, significant amounts of staff
time were being taken up in monitoring her during her visits, and it was
getting to a stage where it was likely that she would be permanently
banned from the site. In addition, she had been caught making racist
comments and gestures towards James, which went against Centre anti-
discrimination policy. Clearly, then, the situation was far less straightforward than it had at first appeared.

At a number of levels I could empathize with the staff. Vandalism and
racism should not be tolerated, whoever the perpetrator happens to be.
Also, it did appear that they had made efforts to resolve the situation with
Vicky and her family so that she could continue to use the Centre, and
that permanent exclusion was very much a final resort when all else had
failed. My main concern about their handling of the situation was in the
way in which they spoke to and about her. It was almost as if, because she

had broken the rules of the Centre, they were then free to do the same, and that as a result of her actions they felt they could speak and behave in ways which they would previously have repressed, as being unprofessional and against the ethos of the Centre. Perhaps in so doing they were actually only revealing what they unconsciously thought of disabled people in general – as being eternal children, requiring surveillance, unable to regulate their own actions – and that other disabled customers only avoided being treated in the same way because they had not broken the rules. Certainly the way that they attempted to infantilize her both through the way they spoke and the judgemental language they used seemed to support social model accounts of the cultural use of negative labelling and terminology as a means of exercising social control over people with learning difficulties (Gelb, 1987). In addition, the series of incidents I observed involving Vicky and the staff acted as a frightening reminder of how fragile the veneer of social engagements between situationally-oppressed and non oppressed people can suddenly become, if the oppressed party transgresses the boundaries as she had done here.

Limitations imposed by the staff role

For members of minority groups, the need to conform to socially acceptable forms of behaviour can be a particularly important survival mechanism, as Vicky found out to her cost. In my own case, the most difficult aspect of being seen as a member of staff was that I was unable to challenge, immediately and publicly, cases of discriminatory practice among non-disabled customers, in case this in turn led to the termination of my field-work. The most blatant and oft-repeated example of such practice was in the routine misuse of accessible disabled-only parking spaces at the Centre. On almost every visit, while I was loading or unloading my chair from the car, a fit-looking non-disabled person would pull up alongside, leap out and run into the building, leaving me fuming in their wake. Sometimes they would even bid me a cheery 'good morning!' or offer to help me put my chair together as they went past – as if that made their actions in parking in these reserved spaces acceptable. Others actually ignored the marked spaces altogether and parked right outside the front door, thus further impeding disabled people's access. Their selfishness and complete lack of awareness of the consequences of their actions was staggering, and the more it happened, the more I absorbed the message that it wasn't just that they felt they had the right to park where they liked, but also that actually in their view disabled people had no right to privileged parking. And at a deeper level, it felt as if by taking those parking spaces they were actually saying 'we don't want you here at all'. In psychoanalytic terms, it might be argued that in such situations the id had temporarily won out over the ego, with the practical outcome that non-disabled people's normally hidden hatred of disabled people (Casling, 1993) was consciously expressed here through denying disabled people the use of the accessible parking bays. This, then, may be seen as another practical example of the persistent day-to-day psychological abuse with which disabled people have to contend (MacFarlane, 1994).

Equally difficult to deal with on such occasions was the lack of response to the situation by Centre staff, which reinforced the catch-22 situation into which I had fallen by working there. At the start of the research, aware that parking was a problem area, James had suggested that my car (minus blue badge) be left in one of the accessible bays and clamped, to act as a visible deterrent to illegal parking. I had previously seen this strategy used to good effect in some supermarket car parks, and was keen to try it out here. However, it somehow came about that each time I asked for it to be done, either the clamp or the key could not be found, and so it never happened. Furthermore, despite my regular complaints, on only one occasion, when the disabled car park was completely full and mine was the only car there which was displaying a blue badge, were the other registration numbers taken and people asked to move their vehicles. This was a sharp reminder both of the limits of my influence in the setting, and of the relative priorities of the Centre. It seemed clear that they were more anxious not to risk upsetting some non-disabled customers by asking them to move their cars than they were to ensure equal access for disabled people. As such this case might be seen as an example of institutional discrimination (Home Office, 1999). In this type of situation, the introduction of structural changes to enforce parking regulations would seem to provide the only solution. However, without overall government legislation to this effect, it is hard to see how individual organizations can be persuaded to ensure equality of opportunity in this way.

Although I did not succeed in persuading the organization to enforce its parking policy in the short term, over time I found that other individual disabled customers – assuming from my frequent presence at the site that I was indeed a member of staff – began reporting other access barriers to me. In these cases I was freed up to take more effective action because they were customer complaints which required an organizational response, lest they should decide to take their business elsewhere. However, it was often apparent that telling me their concerns was a last resort, after previous complaints to management had – so they told me – gone unacknowledged. Sometimes the combination of internal and external pressure did have an effect, as when the shower in one of the accessible changing rooms was fixed. However, in general there seemed to be a gap between the Centre's policy on priority repair work, and its practice. Nor were disabled customers the only ones to feel excluded. A number of staff told me that their own reports of access barriers to management had been similarly ignored, and were all too aware of the negative effect on the Centre's image of its failure to respond to complaints in a timely way. In partial defence of the management, it must be said that all of the access issues raised were targeted in an action plan, which was due to be implemented when the general Centre refurbishment took place. However, junior staff and customers had not been told about this, and so the discontent rumbled on.

Some conclusions

As the examples given in this chapter show, my identity as a member of Greenways staff proved to be a problematic one. On the one hand, my presence at the site as a visible person with impairments increased the impression that the Centre was inclusive and open to everyone, and in turn this may have encouraged some other disabled people to use the facilities. Certainly this did appear to be the case in the gym, where I observed at least four other disabled people starting to work out during the course of the research. In addition, I was able to gain privileged access to members of the management team, and to make suggestions for access improvements which – if not implemented immediately – were at least incorporated into the refurbishment action plan.

On the other hand, I was all too aware both of the limitations of my individual influence on the Centre, and of the fact that at times my presence could be read as sanctioning existing exclusionary practice of which I disapproved. Perhaps such ethical dilemmas are an integral part of any research project which is personally involving. Equally, part of the problem may have been that previously as an access consultant I had been used to going into settings and making recommendations for change, without staying around long enough to see if those changes were actually implemented. Here my long-term presence, and the conflation of my consultant's identity with that of member of staff, revealed that action was not always taken on advice given, which also seemed to confirm wider staff complaints of not being listened to. Whichever of my identities had the most impact in the setting, a catch-22 situation was revealed. At times my staff identity gave me access to staff views and behaviour which they might not have revealed to an outsider consultant, but equally – if my observations of other staff-management relationships were accurate – it may have made managers less ready to act on my suggestions than they might have done had I been a regular paid consultant. The tensions and potential conflicts between these roles were factors which I was never able to satisfactorily resolve in the course of the fieldwork.

In the next chapter I discuss some of the ways in which the friendships I formed at Greenways affected and informed my research. I show how, as the fieldwork progressed, I chose to discuss more openly some personal issues around disability and impairment with my friends there, thereby challenging the injunction of social model thinkers such as Finkelstein and Oliver against the public discussion of such 'private concerns' (Thomas, 1999). I also discuss the effects which adopting this approach had on the research process.

Chapter 7

Being a friend

Pitfalls and opportunities of fieldwork friendships

Before the start of the fieldwork, I had neither expected nor intended to form real friendships with anyone at Greenways. A combination of my old reserved consultant persona and the messages I had drawn from traditional ethnographic research textbooks made me feel it would be better to as far as possible hold myself aloof from the participants while I was there. In part this was a specific response to Hammersley and Atkinson's warning (1983: 72–3) about the potential pitfalls of the researcher's relationship with the site gatekeeper, which needs to be 'good enough' to ensure ongoing access, without becoming so close that the researcher is steered into particular networks of pre-existing friendships and enmities, and towards certain areas of research at the expense of others. At the outset I was unsure of how well I would be able to deal with such potential conflicts, and thus decided that the best course of action would be to remain as detached and uninvolved as possible in my dealings with people at the site.

In the event, however, it was not long before I realized that I could not, and in fact did not want to, pursue this strategy. Two factors influenced this decision. First, as discussed in previous chapters, Greenways was in general a friendly setting, where staff and customers enjoyed a chat and a laugh rather than concentrating solely on perfecting 'the body beautiful'. In these circumstances, it would have looked odd if I had not joined in with some of the friendly banter that went on. Indeed, it might have made it harder to get to know people and to find out their views, had I kept myself to myself. Second, at the time when I started the fieldwork I was also reading Coffey's researcher guide to ethnographic fieldwork relationships, which offered more reassurance about the inevitability of the researcher's involvement in the setting than the books I had previously come across. In particular, as the fieldwork developed I was guided by her statement that:

The primary task of the fieldworker is to analyse and understand a peopled field. This task is achieved through social interaction and shared experiences. It follows, therefore, that fieldwork is dependent upon and guided by the relationships that are built and established over time.

(1999: 39)

Being 'allowed' in this way to accept the need for fieldwork relationships as a means of carrying the research process forward enabled me to relax a little, which in turn probably made me more approachable. Certainly over time I came to chat and share a joke with many staff and customers, and in some cases such interactions led onto the development of real friendships.

The gatekeeper as a friend

Of all my friendships at Greenways, that with James the gatekeeper was the most significant, both in itself, and in its effect on how other people at the site perceived me. From the first meeting onwards, it was clear that we had a similar approach to equality issues, and a shared understanding of oppression which meant we were often able to talk in shorthand, as here:

J: . . . It's a bit like someone saying to me about 'what it's like to be black', as 'what it's like to be disabled' . . . well, I don't know any other way.
C: Exactly.
J: So, that question is, like, a legitimate question from another point of view . . .
C: Yeah, but personally it's meaningless, isn't it?
J: That's right, yes.

Further examples of the similarities in our experiences as a disabled person and a black person are given in Chapter 9, and lend support to previous social model analyses of the links between disablism and racism (Banton and Hirsch, 2000; Borthwick, 1996; Priestley, 1995; Vernon, 1996, 1999). For now, it is important to acknowledge the practical benefits for me in having somebody else at the site who understood from the inside both some of the issues I was dealing with in this research, and why I felt that I needed to do it at all. It was a great relief not to have to explain or justify my approach in the same detail as might have been required in order to convince a white non-disabled gatekeeper of the validity of the research.

From what James has told me, I know that he learned a lot from our work together. For example, although from the outset he displayed a certain awareness of my personal support needs, he also thought that I would want to do as much as possible for myself. This was because his only previous experience of working with disabled people had been with Para-lympic athletes who expected to be given equal access to facilities that they could then use independently. However, I was different in that my level of impairment is such that I no longer waste a lot of time trying to do every-thing for myself, but instead ask whoever I happen to be with at the time to give me a hand. Thus, as Morris has previously argued (1993: 22–4), for me independence is less a matter of being able to do everything for myself, than of choosing how and by whom any necessary support is given.

When I started the fieldwork, however, I was careful not to reveal this philosophy to the participants, because I wanted to see what they would do when faced with a situation where they could see that I might need help. The first time I met James we went for a coffee, and he immediately said that he would get the drinks machine moved so that in future I would be able to reach it more easily and so serve myself. When I said that wasn't necessary because I would always need help with that task from someone else, he was so shocked by the realization that I wasn't even going to try to do it myself that he literally stepped backwards. Then a couple of weeks later we had a confrontation in front of other staff over his refusal to help me sign in one day when I could not reach across to the far page of the Contractors Book to do so myself. Eventually he caved in when I pointed out how bad it would look if the building went up in flames and I was still inside because nobody knew I was there.

At the time I deeply resented such normalizing tendencies on his part, and what felt like an attempt to undermine my whole approach to managing the effects of my impairment. In fact I was so distressed by it that I even con-sidered ditching the research altogether, because I couldn't face the thought of having to battle constantly to justify myself. Eventually what saved the situation was that during a formal interview three months into the study he finally admitted to having some concerns about when and how he should offer me support. Realising that his previous approach had been based on concern rather than a desire to police and normalize my behaviour came as a relief to me, although it was equally important that he now under-stood that I had experienced it as inappropriate. We then had a discussion about how to balance support with autonomy, after which there were no more misunderstandings. However, it was a valuable lesson to both of us. For myself, I realized that although to begin with I had not wanted to be too open about my willingness to receive help, until I gave explicit permis-sion for this to happen even relatively enlightened non-disabled people like him were too scared to take the initiative themselves, for fear of offending me or making it look as if they thought I wasn't capable of performing par-ticular tasks. For him, it was about recognizing that not all disabled people are the same, and that accepting support to save unnecessary time and effort is a sign of strength rather than weakness.

All in all, my friendship with James was extremely important, not just for the fieldwork but for my life in general at that time. Back then I was feeling rather jaded and cynical about the future, and the research experience gave me the mental shake-up I needed to see that I could take more control over what came next. So I will always be grateful to him for his support over those months. Within the setting as a whole it is also likely, as I suggested in the previous chapter, that staff perceptions of our friendship affected how they in turn responded to me. As he himself said, whether they saw me as one of his staff or as his friend, the assumption of a link between us meant that most were careful to act in an inclusive way around me, for fear of negative repercussions otherwise. I am sure that this was true up to a point, although equally I did witness or was on the receiving end of some exclusionary behaviour by staff, as previous examples have shown, so I do not believe that I received a completely sanitized version of events as a result of my links with him. In protecting the integrity of the research, it was also important that I did not – as I know he would have liked – name and shame staff who broke the rules, in case this suggested that I was indeed reporting back verbatim to him. As time went on, however, and none of the staff received negative feedback from him about their reactions to the research, I think they were reassured that I was maintaining a proper code of confidentiality. This in turn led them to trust me more, and to reveal more information.

Greenways as 'a family'

Early on in my research James referred to Greenways as being 'like a family' where people looked out for each other. Certainly observation of general interactions suggested a friendly and inclusive setting where people felt at home. For example, in talking about 'her' customers, one in-house instructor commented:

> they're like a little extension of my family. Because they're not just people from . . . we meet up sometimes, and we'll have a night out, or go for a coffee, sit and chat here, and they become friends as well.

As an individual user of Centre facilities, I soon came to appreciate the protective family atmosphere of the place, where people would appear as if from nowhere to provide me with help and support when needed. One time I was having real trouble explaining to a new receptionist who I was, and was about to resort to writing down what I wanted to say when my friend Sarah materialized beside me and fell unquestioningly into an inter-preter role, easing the situation immediately. Often, too, both staff and customers would open doors for me, or help me with my jacket, always providing such support in low-key ways as one friend will do for another. As such, Greenways quickly became a comfortable and supportive setting for me, and the increase in the amount of friendly teasing to which I soon became subject seemed to indicate that I was becoming an accepted part of the scene. Over time, we achieved a level of trust such that some people were also freed up to laugh with me about the effects of my impairment. For example, when I explained to somebody that I didn't like swimming because of my tendency to go into spasm and sink, he replied that this was good because if I ended up on the bottom of the pool they could turn me into a water feature to scare small children. I never found comments like this offensive, because of the context and the spirit in which they were intended – and because needless to say I could give as good as I got. In fact, such exchanges were a mark of the progress we had made towards having ordinary relationships, rather than ones where people were constantly on tenterhooks in case they said something about my impairment that they thought might offend me.

However, families are not always without their problems, and there were aspects of life at Greenways which I found difficult to deal with. In particular, there was a real culture of gossip and of surveillance which meant that few actions went unobserved, making it both harder and at the same time even more important to maintain confidentiality of the fieldwork data. Some people voiced hopes that I would tell them what others had said in their interviews, or would ask me outright what I had been talking to so-and-so about for such a long time. Occasionally, when I was seen talking to a man, there was also a hint that they thought there was more going on than just an interview. Although this was never actually the case, it was important for me to bear their sensitivities in mind, and to ensure that I was seen not to be doing anything which could make people suspect my motives, and which might in turn jeopardize the integrity of the research.

Friendships with customers

In the course of the fieldwork I also developed friendships with members of some of the contractor-run disability sports groups at the Centre. These relationships tended to be qualitatively different from those with most of the staff, in that they were based on certain shared in-group assumptions to which non-disabled people do not have access. Thus, to begin with, my use of a support worker was a key to my acceptance by the groups as 'one of them'. Frequently too, where I was a wheelchair user and they were not, and if they also knew that I was a researcher when they were not, their superior walking ability acted to help equalize the relationship between us. As a result I quickly became absorbed into a network of close and supportive relationships in which group members revealed their intelligence to each other and to me, but often kept their awareness hidden from the staff, who from their actions seemed unlikely to be prepared to take such displays of intelligence at face value. Thus, for example, one woman would often give me a detailed observational analysis of staff and group behaviour, but as soon as one of the staff came within earshot she would either become silent or would 'go stupid' (Sinason, 1992: 8) by adopting a falsely ingratiating manner and immediately reporting to them that she was 'just helping Claire'. When we were on our own she also frequently sought reassurance that I would not reveal anything she was telling me to the staff, for fear of possible repercussions and retaliation.

To a great extent I could understand why group members behaved in this way. In explaining similar behaviour among people she worked with, Sinason has drawn parallels between the experiences of disabled people and black people:

> some handicapped people behave like smiling pets for fear of offending those they are dependent on. This can involve cutting their real language and intellectual abilities. This type of secondary handicap also has wider political application. When people depend for their lives on cruel regimes they need to cut their intelligence and awareness. Black slaves and their descendants in the USA learned to show their intelligence in private and adopt a 'stupid' appeasing way of talking in front of whites.
>
> (ibid.: 21)

At one level, then, hiding what they knew was a defence against an oppressive regime. It may also have been a symptom of what Swain (1993: 158–9) has called 'learned helplessness', resulting from the knowledge that, whatever their individual hopes and aspirations might have been, most decisions about the course of their lives would continue to be taken by (usually) non-disabled professionals. More positively, it could also be seen as a sort of secret weapon, in that understanding the power relations at work in the 'helper–helped' relationship, without the authorities knowing how much they knew, also allowed for the possibility of resistance. Such a strategy was necessary here because routinely I observed – and was myself on the receiving end of – patronizing and exclusionary behaviour by some of their group leaders. Sometimes in fact it appeared that the sessions at Greenways were organized more for the benefit of those staff than for the groups themselves (see Chapters 11 and 13 for more detailed discussions of this point). In those circumstances, resistance – even at a basic level of becoming mute and letting everything wash over them – was an essential survival mechanism. It may also be argued that sometimes it is both easier and safer to stay locked into particular forms of submissive behaviour than to break the pattern and to begin to take more personal responsibility for our actions by revealing to others the true extent of our capabilities (Symington, 1992: 136). Yet at another level such a strategy was 'a mad defence'

(Sinason, 1992: 137) because it both reinforced stereotyped notions of group members' incompetence in the minds of the staff (Wolfensberger, 1992), and offered no real possibility for members to move forward towards greater independence and self-expression.

In fact while working with the groups I noticed a lot of practical support mechanisms in operation between the members, much of which again went unacknowledged by the staff, except where the intervention of a group member saved them from having to take action themselves. Once someone spilled coffee over herself, and it was another group member who went to get a cloth to mop her up. Another time I saw a man looking so bored and distressed that he had reverted to repetitive rocking behaviour. Again, it was other members of the group who, noticing this, went over and sat quietly talking to him, offering reassurance until his distress eased. Such support mechanisms were also made available to me when I was working with them. For example, while playing hockey with one group of people with learning difficulties, I noticed that several people were taking it upon themselves to deliberately place the ball where I could hit it, even if this meant physically preventing others from taking their shot. When moving between activities, I also regularly found someone behind me, pushing my chair. Sometimes they would ask my permission beforehand, sometimes not. Although I hate it when non-disabled people push me without asking first, here accepting the help of other disabled people without question was crucial, especially because I knew that few of them would have much opportunity to take on responsibility in other areas of their lives, even though they were probably able to do so. Putting my trust in them to get me safely from A to B was a small but important way of showing them that I knew what they were capable of.

For their part, I am sure that sometimes their offers of help were based on mainstream normalizing assumptions about wheelchair users being less capable than other disabled people, and that they wanted to be seen 'helping me'. Perhaps, though, such perceptions are unsurprising given the impact of normalization/SRV programmes on people with learning difficulties, as part of which they may be encouraged to mix primarily with non-disabled people, and to view people with visible impairments as being less capable of 'passing' than those without (Dowse, 2001; Goffman, 1990). However, one distinction remained between their behaviour and that of non-disabled people holding negative views on people with physical impairments. Even where they clearly saw me as being in need of their support, they did not give this in a patronizing way, but in an understated manner designed to include me without fuss in whatever activity was taking place. This was in contrast to the behaviour of some of their non-disabled activity leaders, who seemed to need to make a big fuss in order that everyone would notice how generous they were being in helping me. That the group's inclusive behaviour towards me took place against a backdrop of relationships with their instructors which were often extremely negative and in which they were themselves routinely patronized or ignored, made me appreciate their resilience and friendship all the more.

Some conclusions

In general, my experiences at Greenways seemed to support Coffey's claim that fieldwork can only proceed and develop through the network of the relationships that evolve between the researcher and the participants (1999: 39). Had I kept to my original plan of holding myself aloof from such involvement I feel sure that I would not have been able to uncover the same level of complexity in people's constructions of disability as was eventually possible here. Having said that, it was also true that becoming more involved with participants in the setting did necessitate careful juggling of personal and research priorities at times, and that it was particularly important for me to be seen to be acting as an impartial observer and not as a management spy. By and large I feel that my approach was successful in this respect.

What the research also showed, however, was the limited extent to which Greenways could be described as an inclusive, family setting. As the previous section indicates, through my friendships with some of the disabled people who visited Greenways as part of segregated groups I found that they were sometimes treated in exclusionary and abusive ways by the contract staff who ran their sessions, rather than as valued customers and friends, as was my own experience as an individual visitor to the site. To repeat one of the conclusions of Chapter 5, I suspect that this was mainly because those contractors were not directly accountable to the same equal opportunities policies as were Greenways' own staff. Consequently, it may only be once Greenways staff take over the running of those sessions, or the contractors are required to comply fully with the Centre's ethos and policies in order to retain their teaching slots, that things will change. In the meantime, many disabled people will unfortunately continue to miss out on the benefits of this friendly, relaxed and largely inclusive setting.

Following Thomas' argument that disability is a socially created tool of oppression used against people with impairments in the same way that patriarchy is a socially created tool of oppression used against women (Thomas, 1999), in the next chapter I focus on service provision for women customers at Greenways, and assess some similarities and differences in organizational responses towards women and disabled people.

Chapter 8

Being a woman

Although the main focus of my research was on constructions of disability, during my time at Greenways I also took note of some aspects of the organization's approach to gender equality. This was because I wanted to find out how its policies on providing access for both women and men compared with those on providing access for both disabled and non-disabled people. In the process I soon discovered that there were also wider issues around sexuality and self-representation in the setting which I had not anticipated, and which I needed to take into account in further uncovering both individual and organizational constructions of disability.

Gender and staffing

In analysing the general effectiveness of Greenways' equal opportunities policies in relation to women, I started off by checking the distribution of women and men in jobs across the organization. This review showed that, although at senior and middle management level there was a fairly equal representation of men and women (senior: four men, two women; middle: two men, four women), and in the gym there were three women and two men, in most other areas of work there was evidence of a strong gendering of roles. Eighteen out of the twenty-four lifeguards were men, as were six out of the nine customer service staff (whose jobs involved a lot of equipment-moving), and all three maintenance workers. On the other hand, all nine receptionists, all three crèche workers, and nearly all the catering and cleaning staff were women. In policy terms there was a stated commitment to equal opportunities for women employees, but this analysis of actual staffing ratios suggested room for improvement, including perhaps the provision of childcare for staff, particularly where their hours of work included antisocial hours; and the need to address gender imbalances in all areas of work below management level. In terms of service delivery, reversing such imbalances would also be an important way of ensuring a fairer mix of activities on offer to customers. One manager had already realized this, in deciding to have female-dominated leadership of future holiday play schemes so as to increase the range of activities provided, and, as she put it, to make it less likely that football would be the only activity on offer to the children.

Service provision for women customers

Conversations with the staff revealed that up to about five years ago most of the leisure activities on offer at Greenways had been segregated into women-only and men-only days, primarily in order to provide safe spaces for women to participate in sport without being watched by men. However, as one manager explained, things have now changed:

> Originally we were trying to get women back into leisure and sport, which 5, 6, 7 years ago, yes. But leisure is such a big thing now, everybody in the world does it, and I don't think it's as much for women to say 'oh, I couldn't go and do that' . . . (previously) we were ideal to get women to come into our Centre, and use it and see that it's not so male-dominated . . .

This comment was representative of the views of a number of Greenways' female staff, who felt that in general women were now confident enough to access the facilities in mixed sessions. This seemed to be supported by a customer survey which showed that in one month in 2000 more than twice as many women as men (70 per cent to 30 per cent) used the Centre. The organization had seemingly taken account of the ongoing nature of such confidence-building both in its staffing and activity programming. For example, one middle-aged woman member of staff reported that some of the older women customers preferred having people like her on duty because they felt they could have a chat and discuss their body shapes with less embarrassment than might have been the case with the younger staff. More formal measures to ensure equal opportunities had also been taken. One morning a week was still reserved as women-only, when in addition to being able to use the main facilities at a reduced rate, they could also join in with targeted fitness activity sessions like 'body conditioning', and 'resistance, circuits and stretch'. Such activities were supplemented with information and advice sessions specifically on women's health issues, and were occasionally further supported by visits from the local Women's Health Bus.

At one level such sessions could be seen as part of the wider social pressure on women to aspire to 'the body beautiful' (Glassner, 1992), and it was undoubtedly true that some of the women I observed week after week in these sessions had wonderful figures and were in great shape. However, for others, taking part was clearly an effort – if also a lot of fun. Observation of a range of the women taking part in these sessions suggested that, while getting fit was part of the deal, for many of them the social aspect of being out in the community and meeting people was equally important. For example, a number of the older women I met were either widowed or were single and had retired from work, and they told me that having somewhere to go like Greenways was crucial to avoiding loneliness and increasing their sense of well-being. Such data would seem to challenge those sociological accounts which claim that everyone in Western cultures today is uncritically obsessed with 'the body project' for its own sake (Giddens, 1991), and suggests the need to develop more holistic explanations for why people choose to take exercise. I return to this point in Chapter 10.

Despite the positive experiences reported above, however, it would be misleading to suggest that the setting was a wholly inclusive one for all non-disabled women. Over the timescale of the research I observed less than ten black women, and no Asian women at all, using the facilities. Staff reported the impossibility of providing segregated swimming sessions for those Asian women who needed them in what was a completely open-plan swimming area, and said that most segregated sports sessions for these women took place at another Centre, where the pool had been designed to allow for this. However, although I asked, no explanation could be given for the lack of minority ethnic women using the gym during the women-only sessions. I was left with the uneasy feeling that the Centre had not seen the need to attract women from minority ethnic groups because there was deemed to be suitable provision elsewhere in the town.

In a few cases, too, sexism was uncovered as people tried to avoid being racist, as here, when a situation at another Centre was being described:

> they had a half day for women only, and a lot of men kicked up about it and said 'that's sexist' and all the rest of it, and 'we want a men's day', but then it was pointed out to them the only reason is that Asian women won't – cannot – train or swim with a male instructor. And then they kind of – a lot of them – 'well, if that's the reason then that's OK'. It's not just a women's thing that 'we want to be separate'.

Since the male member of staff who told me this made no attempt to qualify or to distance himself from the sentiments expressed in this statement, I concluded that he probably sympathized with such views about calls for segregated provision being a separatist 'women's thing'. For some staff, then, it seemed that segregated provision was only to be tolerated on religious, cultural or impairment grounds, and not solely on the basis of gender, even though Greenways as an organization recognized the ongoing need for some women-only sessions to raise confidence levels among any or all of the women customers. Taken together, these observations suggested underlying racism and sexism in the setting, and the need to develop more effective anti-discrimination measures to make the Centre's approach to service provision truly inclusive.

Sexuality at Greenways

The issue of sexuality first came to the fore during my access negotiations with James, when he made it clear that I would not be allowed to take any photographs at Greenways 'because people don't always come here with the right partners'. Clearly staff were used to this sort of occurrence, just as in countryside recreation we would sometimes have to look the other way if we came across courting couples during site patrols. Perhaps it is a general issue for people who work in recreation settings, needing to be aware that some of their customers may take the concept of rest and relaxation further than others! In any case, over time I became increasingly aware of the Centre – especially the pool area – as a sexualized space for a number of the customers. For example, there were the teenage boys playing with a toy whale, making it spout water in what seemed to be a simulation of masturbation, and then collapsing in fits of knowing laughter; while another day I couldn't get into the accessible/disabled changing room because it was occupied by two women who appeared to have been having sex.

At the same time, however, there seemed to be little positive recognition of disabled people's sexuality in the setting. For example, the women-only sessions described above took place at the same time that one of the disability groups – comprising both men and women – used the Centre. Yet nobody seemed to see this as odd or inappropriate, leading me to the conclusion that this form of mixed provision was acceptable because the disabled men present were seen as safe and/or asexual. In fact the issue of disabled people's sexuality was one on which several otherwise politically correct people at the Centre betrayed less inclusive inner thoughts. For example, once I was discussing with a friend the actions of a disabled man who had asked me out. I said I thought his sometimes frighteningly direct and persistent style was at least in part due to the lack of a general sex education for disabled people in schools and day centres, so that he simply hadn't been taught how to approach a woman and ask her out. She agreed, but then as our discussion continued she referred to him unthinkingly as 'a lad'. When I corrected her, and said that actually I thought he was about our age (late thirties), she shivered suddenly and said that made her feel sick. It seemed that while she could 'other' him by thinking of him as being much younger than her she could cope with the idea of his sexuality, and the fact that he had not yet learned to express it appropriately. Realising that he was our age – was perhaps 'like us' – and had unfulfilled sexual feelings was harder to deal with. In part I think this was because it brought home to her more clearly the fact that disabled people are not always properly supported in ways that would enable them to explore and express their sexuality. However, it is possible that another reason for her reaction may have been related to more deep-rooted unconscious social fears that indicate a preference to keep the sexuality of people with learning difficulties suppressed (Chappell, 1998; Wolfensberger, 1992). In this context, discovering that disabled people have sexual needs in the same way that non-disabled people do may also threaten non-disabled people's assumptions that they are different from, and in this respect superior to, disabled people.

Being a woman researcher

For myself, I know that my self-image as a woman improved considerably during the research, and that this development was also closely bound up with the friendships I made and a growth in fitness and self-confidence (as discussed further in Chapter 10). As I began to find my way around and to be recognized as an accepted part of the scene, so I felt more comfortable with a high public visibility that I would previously have shunned. In the process I began to lose some of my former self-consciousness, and, as other people made it clear that they found me attractive, to discover and own my own sexuality. For the first time in my life it felt OK to adopt the labels of 'woman' and 'sexual being' without adding an ironic comment to play down my effrontery at calling myself a real woman. In short, I was coming to feel happier with the whole of who I am. In more formal research terms, I was also aware that my identity as a woman was sometimes a key to reassuring other women that it was safe to take part, especially during the interview phase of the project (Finch, 1993; Ozga and Gewirtz, 1994). This commonality helped me to provide a supportive environment in which they could safely express their fears and concerns about disability and impairment, issues which most admitted they had never discussed with a disabled person before. As a result of taking this approach I am aware that several of the interview transcripts with members of staff read more like gossipy chats than formal research data, but I make no apology for this, because the effect of trying to put people at ease in this way was to at least sometimes enable honest and in-depth discussions of their thoughts on these issues. However, the conflation of my researcher identity with those of being both a woman and a disabled person in the interview situation made it even more important that I gave all of the interviewees a copy of their transcript, in case they felt that they had become too relaxed, and had revealed more of their thoughts and feelings to me than they had intended. I was also aware that I probably conducted many of my interviews with men in a slightly different way than in those with the women, taking deliberate advantage of my gender to present myself to the men as non-threatening and sympathetic (Ozga and Gewirtz, 1994: 121), in order that they would open up to me. However, this had mixed results. Sometimes men who had previously been approachable and helpful before and during the interview became more distant once I had given them their transcripts. This may have been because they then realized that they had actually said more than they meant to during our discussions, although none went so far as to then withhold permission for me to use their data in the research. In other cases, though, men became more friendly and helpful after the interview, giving the impression that they had valued what we had shared during our discussion. Consequently I would not wish to draw any firm conclusions on the presence and effect or otherwise of gendered reactions to the interviews conducted for this research.

Some conclusions

The data discussed in this chapter have revealed something of the influence of gender and sexuality on service provision within the setting. Although there was some evidence of sexism, it was also a place where I regularly saw men taking their children swimming, and openly lavishing care and love on them. Clearly for them the Centre was a safe space in which they could unselfconsciously express their love for their children in ways that might not have been encouraged within other public settings. Once more, then, the data showed up a mass of contradictions and the possibility of there being any number of different 'takes' on what was going on at Greenways, and how people saw and responded to each other. It also suggested further limits to the effectiveness of the Centre's current equalities policies, both in terms of the gendering of many jobs below management level, and in the knock-on effect that such gendering might on occasion have for the sorts of services offered to customers.

In terms of helping to uncover constructions of disability in the setting, the comparison undertaken between service provision for women and disabled customers was useful in that it revealed both similarities and differences in approaches to provision for the two groups. In terms of similarity, value was attached to segregated provision as a means of developing skills and confidence levels among both groups. However, a major difference was also apparent, in that most site provision for white non-disabled women was inclusive, with only one half-day of segregated activities on offer, whereas most provision for disabled people was through segregated groups, with relatively few being observed to visit the Centre independently. Economics may have been an additional complicating factor here, in that many of the disabled customers did not have jobs, and thus may have had no option but to join in the subsidized segregated group activities. In terms of Centre policy, one positive development arising out of this project has been the extension of the existing subsidized pricing policy to include the offer of discounted admission prices to disabled people. This should give disabled people more opportunity to participate in mainstream sessions in the future. However, as later chapters will discuss in more detail, interviews with staff also seemed to suggest that they had no real expectation that segregated group members, most of whom were people with learning difficulties, would be able to participate alongside non-disabled people in this way. The main reasons given for this were a perceived lack of physical ability and/or a perceived need for the provision of extra support. The main difference in approach, then, was that for people with learning difficulties segregated provision was seen as the most appropriate leisure option, whereas for white women it was only one of a range of accepted means of participation.

As some of the data in this chapter has shown, during the research it also became apparent that the Centre was not always an inclusive space for people from minority ethnic groups. In the next chapter I look at aspects of that experience as it was represented to me. I explore some of the similarities and differences in the experience of exclusion for black people and disabled people, and show what drawing on the whole of that experience helped to reveal about the operation of institutional discrimination within the setting.

Chapter 9

Being white

The relative absence of people from minority ethnic groups from Greenways

As I had done in assessing the extent of women's inclusion at Greenways, so I began this part of the research by looking at the numbers of people from minority ethnic groups employed by the Centre. Despite the Centre's equal opportunities policy, I found that there were only five black and Asian members of staff at Greenways out of the overall staff complement of seventy-two. All five were male, which perhaps reflected the gendering of most non-management posts at the Centre discussed in the previous chapter. Four worked part-time and one was full-time, and only the full-time person (James) was in a management position. From my observation there also seemed to be very few black and Asian customers at the site, with more (especially teenaged boys and girls) participating in sports hall activities such as basketball and football than were present in and around the pool area. Granted, my observations were primarily of daytime visits, when many people would have been at work, and it is quite possible that more people from minority ethnic groups visited the site during the evenings, in line with the general increase in use of facilities like the gym after work. However, staff feedback also supported my view that there was relatively low use of the Centre by people from minority ethnic backgrounds.

More particularly, I only ever saw one minority ethnic disabled person at Greenways, and he was swimming with his family at weekends. No black or Asian disabled people participated in the segregated disability group sessions, all of which were run by departments of the local council. In part there may have been cultural explanations for this, in that 'some Black and ethnic minority people with disabilities and their families might not share the view of their white counterparts that a disabled person has a "right" to certain services and should do their best to exercise such a right' (Banton and Hirsch, 2000: 6). However, assumptions of a preference within minority ethnic communities to 'look after their own' have been questioned by some research (Department of Health, 2001), which has highlighted the need for disability services to promote themselves more effectively across all communities. At present, as Banton and Hirsch point out (2000: 34), many black and Asian disabled people fall between two stools in terms of service provision, being marginalized by white organizations because they are black, and by black organizations because they are disabled people. They stress the importance for all organizations which claim to offer services to black disabled people of changing their procedures, practices and culture to increase accessibility, and offer a wide range of suggestions for practical ways of achieving this (ibid.: 34–41). Although my own research did not look in detail at the reasons for the marginalization of minority ethnic disabled people at Greenways, their lack of representation at the site was reported to the organization, and will be addressed in a future research project.

Evidence of racial stereotyping among Greenways staff

From my conversations with white members of staff at Greenways, it soon became apparent that few were actively aware of the absence of people from minority ethnic groups from the setting. Often when I asked them why they thought there were few minority ethnic members of staff or customers they expressed surprise at the question, and said they hadn't thought about it before. Worryingly, most then offered racist reasons for those absences:

> A: I think a lot of that's to do with culture, the actual culture of the ethnic minorities, and how they view things like work ethic and leisure and play, and I think they tend to have a strong work ethic, and so they put less emphasis and less time towards leisure.

> B: . . . I don't think they don't come here because they're coloured. I think they probably don't come here because it's – they are complicated classes.

> C: . . . in the area that this is, this isn't really, I mean, you do get a few black people, Asians and so . . . but it's not an area where you see a lot of them. The majority of people in this area are white, basically, so I suppose that comes into it.

> D: Black people tend not to apply for poolside jobs because they are either very good swimmers or very poor, and this is related to their physique.

> E: . . . there's the classic thing of the black kid in the class who's going to be good at sprinting and running and strength-oriented activities, because of the build – it's in the genes of that particular race, and

they're more prone to be good at those sports, and so they don't need the same amount of training or work-outs as white people.

These comments reveal the prevalence of stereotyped racist views which tended to blame the victim for their exclusion, and which also showed how minority ethnic groups were constructed in this setting as 'Other'. This finding mirrors that of Bagihole (1997: 174), who reported that previous cultural explanations for ethnic minorities' low take-up of publicly available services have tended to attribute the cause to 'the assumed inadequacy of ethnic minorities themselves and their family formation, thus ignoring structural inequality and past disadvantage'. In both respects, these findings have parallels with the experience of disabled people. Here, it was assumptions about the culture, genes, geographical placement, and 'natural sporting prowess' of people from minority ethnic groups which were held to be responsible for their absence from the site, and not the Centre's failure to attract a more representative cross-section of staff and customers.

For example, it appeared that even – or perhaps particularly – among some of the sports coaches, assumptions about specifically black people's natural sporting ability prevailed, with no account being taken of the wider social and economic factors which can make participation in sport one of the few pathways to success for black people. Sport may be an activity into which they find themselves being pushed by white teachers when they are at school and, as Gillborn explains (1990: 113), this may act as a crude means of social control, 'reflecting and reinforcing crude stereotypes of Afro-Caribbean pupils as more suited to physical/manual tasks than to academic/non-manual ones'. Although they may then do well at sport this might only be because that is the only area open to them to succeed in. However, white staff at Greenways seemed unaware of these complex and potentially problematic aspects of black people's sporting success, instead seeing it in wholly uncomplicated and positive terms. Nor did they see any apparent contradiction between the statement about Greenways being in a mainly white area, and the marketing department's research which showed that the Centre's catchment area covered people living within eight minutes' drive-time, which in effect took in most of the town's multi-ethnic population rather than just specific parts of it. Although one or two people did mention the lack of targeted information provision to minority groups about what Greenways had to offer them as creating a structural barrier to participation, on the whole the absence of minority ethnic people from the setting was seen as 'their own fault'. Uncovering such casually expressed racist sentiments came as a real shock to me. As a result of these findings, one of the recommendations in my final consultancy report was that race equality training should be given to all staff, to encourage them to review their often unconscious racist assumptions and to develop more inclusive practice for the future.

Nor can I avoid reporting my own complicity in perpetuating racism at the site. In many ways, as previously reported, my friendship with James was central to the research. Yet it is painful to have to admit that it was only after the fieldwork had ended, and I was reading more widely around some of the issues raised, that I consciously acknowledged both the impact which my being white must have had on our relationship, and the need to foreground this aspect of my identity in my research analysis. In part I feel that this omission came about because, as I will discuss below, our personal connections in terms of our shared experience of oppression were often stronger than the elements that divided us. Still, I must admit that for me, my own whiteness was throughout much of the research an invisible, un-contested category (hooks, 2000: 56; Giroux, 1992: 116–7; Wong, 1994: 136), and that there were times when as a white researcher I could have been accused of perpetuating racism by neither seeing nor challenging it (Trepagnier, 1994; Vernon, 1999: 389–90).

Race and impairment – some differences and connections

Although few in number, some non-disabled black people did use Green-ways, and I got to speak to several black women during the daytime sessions. Each time this happened I was struck by a feeling of connection between us, with two incidents in particular springing to mind. One day I had just parked the car and was putting my chair together when two black women, one older and one thirty-ish and walking with a stick, came out of the Centre. Seeing me putting the handles on my chair, the older woman came over and offered to help, so I let her take over. As she finished she said 'It's the little things sometimes, isn't it?'. We all laughed, and then they went on their way. It was one of those brief moments of shared experience and understanding when you feel relieved that you don't have to explain everything all the time. And then the second time I was struggling to open a heavy door when a young black woman came along and gave me a hand. We were laughing about it, and I told her how I'd got stuck in the same doorway the week before and had to wait to be rescued, and she said 'I think they make them heavy on purpose'. I assumed that she meant 'to keep you/us out'. Once more, it felt like a moment of understated awareness and solidarity. Both incidents reminded me of Hockenberry's account of his experience as a wheelchair user of trying to use the New York subway for a radio programme he was recording:

> At this point, every white person I had encountered had ignored me or pretended that I didn't exist, while every black person who came upon me had offered to help without being asked. I looked at the tape recorder in my jacket to see if it was running. It was awfully noisy in

the subway, but if any voices at all were recorded, this radio program was going to be more about race than it was about wheelchair accessibility. It was the first moment that I suspected the two were deeply related in ways I have had many occasions to think about since.

(1995: 308)

Having mentioned these points of connection between myself and some of the black women I met, it must also be noted that during the research I came across some cultural barriers which might hinder dialogue between disabled people and people from minority ethnic groups. For example, I have to admit that, although there were five black and Asian members of staff at Greenways, James was really the only one I spoke to during the fieldwork. It wasn't that I didn't try to speak to the others, but each time I did so I found that they avoided my eye and kept going. I have since read (Gillborn, 1990: 37) that among some Afro-Caribbean people turning the eyes away is a sign of deference and respect. However, as a disabled person I had only previously been used to people avoiding my eye out of disgust, and so this was – rightly or wrongly – how I interpreted their behaviour, especially given that the black women I met had no such qualms about meeting my eye. As a result I chose not to follow up the encounters with these men, for fear of further rejection. This, then, is one small example of the cultural and gender confusions which may help perpetuate differences between people from minority ethnic groups and disabled people, and between men and women. With James, too, there were times when I breached unspoken boundaries through my choice of language. Once we were discussing how to improve access to one area of the Centre, and he suggested providing a separate entrance for disabled people to that part of the facility. Without thinking, I immediately protested 'but you can't do that – it would be like apartheid'. His look of shock and anger at my use of language here told me that I had gone too far by hijacking a term inextricably linked to race struggles and using it instead to describe the exclusion of disabled people. However, he obviously took on board the point I was making, if not the way it was expressed, because he never again suggested such an access 'solution'.

Despite the presence of such barriers and misunderstandings, the points of connection which developed in particular between James and me were crucial to the development of the research. One of the most shocking of all my discoveries at Greenways was the realization that although he was a high-level manager and something of a sporting celebrity, he still faced the same sorts of prejudice and oppression as the rest of us. Naively, I had hoped to find that there was some point of personal success beyond which people from minority groups could find protection from discrimination, and discovering that this would never be the case was a real blow. However, at the same time as recognizing the general inflexibility of wider society, we found we could still discuss and develop strategies for change which might make a difference, if only in small ways. In this extract from one of our interviews, James highlights some of the similarities in our experience, and offers some suggestions for moving forward:

C: Right, so what similarities are there between black people's and disabled people's experience?
J: Always having to fight for things that everyone else gets as a matter of course. Having to justify why you want something. Having to be seen to be better than your colleagues, even though people tell you that you've no need to. Having to be used as a 'shining example' all the time, as someone who's achieved something from way down the bowels of the earth. (Laughter) And there's a little bit of toleration, I suppose, of the work that you've done. It's always 'unique', always 'something we'll get our expert to do'. Always to be seen as an expert. And also, there is that element of 'thou shalt not go past' a certain level. Now that level may or may not be reached at this stage, but it's justified to do it, because you're always marked. Because the better you are around the system, in terms of academic or whatever, then people know you, know your type, and know where you're going to fit in. It's like, if you applied for a post now, the name, unusual as it is, won't be seen as someone who's a researcher – but it'll be someone who's in – as a wheelchair user, and that will go round like wildfire, which again I don't like. And also I think that mainstream pick you out as their champion for disadvantage, and disabled users, for example, automatically gravitate to you, but I don't want them to. I don't want black members of the public trying to say hello to me – I don't need it. You are using the facility and that's it . . .
C: How can we get beyond that – or d'you think we can?
J: It is very difficult, because we're the one that's pushing, and as such we're the one that's experiencing it, and that needs to be out to say 'speak to me, but don't speak at me'. If you've got a problem then I'll deal with it, but I don't want to deal with it because I'm in a chair or because I'm black. And I think we need to be pushing out information in the same way that maybe the gay community has, we should learn from the gay community, because I think they've been very open and transparent in how they've conducted – to include the MPs. In the past it was covert – now it's out and like 'so what?' . . .

I found his description of much of our experience – which we had not previously discussed in such detail – unerringly accurate here, and have little to add by way of analysis, other than to agree that we need to get to a position where challenging disadvantage ceases to be the responsibility of individual figureheads within particular organizations, and instead becomes a more general social duty. However, it is also important to note that until we did this interview, in the final month of the fieldwork, I was not aware of the full extent of either our shared experience of discrimination, or of the existence of institutional racism at the site. We had not made these connections explicit, but instead had worked together using a set of unspoken shared assumptions.

Yet an incident a few days later made me realize that maybe this under-stated approach had certain limitations. I was conducting an interview with someone who started by expressing the patronizingly offensive views about disabled people previously reported in Chapter 4. The interviewee then began talking about the employment quota system (Disabled Persons' (Employment) Act 1944), and his belief that this arrangement guaranteed paid work to a good percentage of disabled people. When I explained that the quota system had never worked effectively and had been scrapped under the provisions of the 1995 Disability Discrimination Act, he was outraged. He said that because ordinary non-disabled people like him had heard there was a quota system, they had assumed that disabled people had real opportunities for employment. To find out that this was not the case, and that no such safety net existed, was a genuine shock to him. As we discussed it further, he then asked me how non-disabled people like him could be expected to support disabled people's struggles for equality if we as disabled people did not first share some of our experiences of discrimi-nation with them, so that they could learn about and understand these issues.

At that moment I realized that part of the difficulty disabled people have faced in challenging exclusionary policies and practices has resulted from this simple fact – that disabled people have rarely been in a position to explain to outsiders the limitations of such provision in the way that he was suggesting. This in turn has made it more difficult to develop alliances with other groups who might have been able to support our struggles for reform. Yet on the relatively infrequent occasions that such alliances have developed they can be powerful forces for change, as demonstrated by the coming together in Britain of disabled people, parents and educators united in their commitment to inclusive education. On a smaller scale, in this research if I had not worked with James I would never have been in a position to understand something of the hidden nature of institutional racism at the site, expressed through factors such as lack of a set career development structure for minorities staff, and the fact that, as described in the previous chapter, the building was an exclusionary space for Asian women. Thus in conducting this research I was brought up against the reali-zation that there are times when disabled people, and black people, and members of other minority groups, need to find ways of talking more expli-citly about the oppression we face, as a step towards forming alliances for change with others.

Some conclusions

In this chapter, I have shown something of the existence of racist perspectives at Greenways, and have also highlighted some similarities and differences in the experiences of minority ethnic and disabled people. Overall there appeared to be less leisure provision for minority ethnic groups at the Centre than there was for disabled people, with one community development worker explaining that segregated sessions for Asian women tended to be organized instead in local halls or community centres where access by outsiders could be more strictly controlled. It was reassuring to know that there was at least some such provision in the town, but at the same time it was worrying that there appeared to be no structures in place to support participants in moving on to sessions at all of the mainstream leisure centres if they so wished. The research therefore suggests the need for more consideration to be given by Greenways as to how to provide more services that black and Asian people want, and what additional support – such as segregated sessions, targeted information and transport provision, translation services, and subsidized pricing – might be needed to facilitate this.

In looking to combat the exclusion of disabled people both at Greenways and elsewhere, drawing parallels from the experiences, philosophies and strategies of other excluded groups and forming temporary and situational alliances with them, would seem helpful both in avoiding unnecessary replication of effort, and in presenting a large and united front to those who exclude us all. However, this is not to say that such an approach is unproblematic. My own experience in this setting showed that white disabled people need to be aware that some black people see eye contact as disrespectful, rather than assuming it's just that they can't stand the sight of us (although there is indeed acknowledged stigma of disabled people in some black communities (Banton and Hirsch, 2000: 22)). Equally, all non-disabled people need to be aware of the negative message which lack of eye contact can give to many disabled people. And there are wider sensitivities which we all need to be aware of, as when James reacted with shock and anger when I named the suggestion that disabled people use an alternative entrance to part of the facility as a form of apartheid. Some terms do appear sacred to some groups, and as such need to be afforded proper respect. However, there may also be occasions when we need to push the boundaries in our search for common ground.

Although I have called this chapter 'Being white', I am conscious that throughout much of it I have actually fallen into the trap identified by Charles (1992: 30) of reporting the experience of black people rather than actively questioning my own whiteness and the ways in which I was implicated in supporting existing forms of racist oppression at the site. In part I now realize that, until James explained it to me, I was simply unaware of the structural aspects of that oppression, though not some of the individual expressions of it. More fundamentally, I found it a real struggle to grasp a sense of my whiteness in a setting where most other people were also white. Until that point it had truly been a taken-for-granted category for me, and I cannot really say that I had been actively aware of my status as a member of a majority in that way, perhaps because other aspects of my identity are usually foregrounded. This in turn has led me to reflect that perhaps 'identity' is most important when you belong to a minority whose selfhood is constantly challenged by the presence and actions of a majority. I must now concede that the difficulties I have had in trying to explore my own majority status as white in this setting have given me an unwitting insight into just how hard it must be for non-disabled people to question their own majority status over me as a disabled person. There are some big issues here, to do with how you get people to question something they have always taken for granted, and who are the most appropriate people to help them to do it. Perhaps this is one of the keys to the way forward – that until we start engaging with each other, minorities with minorities and minorities with majorities, we can't start asking questions about those things we thought we knew before. After all, if I hadn't worked with James, I might never have recognized my whiteness as a factor in the research, or noticed how few black and Asian people were present at Greenways, or even have tried to write this chapter. I can now see the limitations of my analysis, and that it's something I need to continue to work on in the future, but I would never have even thought about race and ethnicity as issues for this research if James hadn't started to disrupt my previous cosy assumptions about 'colour-blindness'.

Having in this and the previous chapter looked at some of the differences and similarities between the ways in which sexism, racism and disablism operated at Greenways, I now move on in subsequent chapters to address more overtly 'personal issues', which are particularly linked to my own and other people's experiences of impairment and disability in this setting. I will start by looking at the experience of 'being a body' at Greenways, and at how this related to some of the wider issues around embodiment and its relationship to the emerging sociology of impairment.

Chapter 10

Being a body

Managing my own embodiment in the setting

In Chapter 3 I described the process behind my initial decision to present at Greenways as a regular wheelchair user. Here I want to reflect a bit more on how that decision worked out in practice, and what this in turn taught me about my own embodiment. My first discovery was that I could not isolate my experience at Greenways from what happened to me in other settings, as the following incident shows. Quite early on in the research I realized that I would need to buy some proper work-out gear to wear when I went to the gym, so I went out shopping for this with a friend. On entering the local sports shop, however, we were both struck by the negative way in which the shop assistants treated me. All the young male sales staff averted their gaze as I came near, while the older woman who finally served me kept calling me 'sweetheart' and spoke in a sorrowful tone as if to imply that, though she applauded my spirit in buying sports gear, she saw it as being more or less a waste of time. Had I not needed the clothes in a hurry, I would undoubtedly have taken my business elsewhere, because I can do without that sort of negative reaction. Equally, had I been a less confident person, I might well have absorbed their implicit message that I was a hopeless case, and have given up on the idea of working out in the gym altogether. In the long term, it is likely that only a combination of targeted economic boycotting, compulsory disability equality training for all staff, and the introduction of properly enforceable anti-discrimination legislation, will bring about wholesale change in exclusionary settings like this one. It also shows that it is not enough simply for leisure centres to demonstrate inclusive practice, but that all associated organizations and suppliers will need to do the same. Otherwise it is all too likely that some disabled people will be dissuaded from sporting participation because of negative experiences like the one described here.

My second discovery was fortunately far more positive. Somewhat to my surprise I quickly found that my general fitness levels increased as a result of being at Greenways. Within weeks I was able to open heavy doors that had previously defeated me, and my field notes record that:

> As I work I experience a feeling of deep joy at how much easier I am finding it to push around the place after only three weeks' practice. I spin, I glide, I race in turn, and just feel so glad to be alive, and doing this work here and now . . . and it could get better still. As people turn to watch me shoot past I know I look good in my own terms – their view, whether for good or bad, doesn't matter at all. Hold that thought.

Working at Greenways thus became a time and a space in which I could reclaim and celebrate my body in a way that most other settings preclude. It was a social setting in which I was able to assist new users unfamiliar with the gym equipment, and to receive help from others in turn when I myself got stuck, without any big fuss being made, as was the Greenways way. I loved taking part in sports activities there, and being able to turn off my mind and simply enjoy my physicality. Through my participation, I thus rediscovered the fact that it is necessary to have a space where I can be all of me, and not just a talking head. Another unexpected bonus was the way in which going for a work-out often gave me a space in which to work through issues to do with this research which I was not able to resolve simply by sitting at my computer. For me, then, as for some of the Centre staff and customers:

> Exercise and thought recursively create the possibility for each other, and either without the other is deprived.
>
> (Frank, 1991: 84)

Nor was my participation a mere research tool or passing fad – I continued to work out regularly well after the end of the research.

I also particularly liked the fact that at Greenways I could keep control of the decisions about which sports to participate in, and how far to push myself. Although some of the staff were very goal-orientated, seeing my active involvement as a means of 'beating my impairment' in a way that I found offensive, most were more laid-back. In part I think this was because I was seen as a fellow member of staff, and so they did not feel the need to question my motivation in joining the gym; and it may also have been because most female gym users were seen as just wanting to lose weight before going on holiday, rather than being there to acquire the body beautiful, and that I was seen as no different to anyone else in that respect.

The same message that I was being seen as an ordinary user came across from other women customers, as my increasingly active participation in

Centre activities led to more, and better quality, interactions with them. A couple of weeks after I started using the gym, a number of women started speaking to me as a fellow regular. One commiserated with me about the small changing rooms, and said she always kept the cubicle door open while she was getting changed, so that she had more space. Another said 'Hello, are you going upstairs, or have you been?' and when I said I was on my way up she said 'See you up there, then'. And as I made my way round the equipment that day I saw her again a couple of times, and she mouthed at me 'How's it going?'. Interactions like these made me feel that I was being admitted on equal terms to their community. However, male customers were more reserved, and during the course of the fieldwork none offered me assistance, even in situations where they saw me struggling. This may have been because they felt less confident around me than the women did, or simply because they did not know how to approach me to offer help. These explanations were suggested by my subsequent experience, in that after the fieldwork ended and I continued to use the gym, I found that some of the men did start to say hello and to give me a hand if I needed it. So it seemed it was less that they hadn't wanted to help before, or that they didn't think I should have been there, than that they were either too shy to make the first move, or felt concerned that offering help to a woman might be taken the wrong way.

Interestingly, many of the women who offered me support at Greenways were significantly older than me, perhaps in their sixties or seventies, and were not of an age group that I would instinctively have expected to behave in an inclusive manner towards me. This seemed to point to the conclusion that there is something about having an aim in common that can bring people together, regardless of age, background or appearance. For example, one woman I spoke to was a widow, and she said that Greenways is an important social outlet for her, and that whenever she's asked out she drops everything and goes, rather than staying at home on her own. I said I could relate to that, and she agreed, saying it wouldn't do either of us any good sitting at home by ourselves. At the end of our conversation she then gave me a hand getting my fleece on, as usual without making a fuss about it. Most members of a regular older persons' group at the Centre seemed like her to be single women in their sixties and seventies, although there was at least one couple there as well. Again, none of them batted an eyelid about my impairment. One asked what sports I did, and when I said 'none', she said she'd thought I must be sporty because I had a sports chair – which was observant of her. So I said the chair was sporty, but I wasn't, which raised a laugh. Later I went to have coffee with them, and could only get a new type of straw which had half of it cut away, so it was very difficult to get a seal and suction. Without waiting to be asked, the woman who'd asked about my chair turned the straw the other way up so I could drink at least some of my coffee, and then squashed the end and held it so I could finish it off. Nobody else stared or saw anything unusual in this. Most were grandparents themselves, so I guess they've been around the block a few times and aren't fazed by much, and we had a nice social chat based on our shared experience of using the Centre. On the whole their perceptions of me were expressed in positive rather than patronizing ways, with my impairment being raised by them in terms of whether or not I needed them to do anything to assist my inclusion, rather than because they wanted to take responsibility for me in some way.

Other disabled people's embodiment at Greenways

I soon discovered that I was not the only person with impairments who felt comfortable enough to exercise regularly at Greenways. Some, like me, preferred to participate at relatively quiet times of the day and week, when it was less likely that they would be accidentally bumped or jostled, especially in using the pool. One woman with learning difficulties went swimming at least once a week, and seemed to love shouting out loud in order to hear her voice echoing back to her from the pool walls. Other older women with a range of physical impairments also went swimming alongside their non-disabled friends, many such groups seeming to spend as much time chilling out and gossiping in the adjacent spa pool as they did in serious swimming. Over time as they got to know me some of them tried to persuade me to join in as well, because they enjoyed it so much, but I was never really confident enough of my swimming ability to do so.

Originally I had assumed that most disabled people would use the facilities at quiet times, but events proved that I was mistaken. During busy Sunday morning sessions I regularly saw two identifiable people with impairments – one the parent of two small children, the other a young girl – in the crowded pool as part of their wider family groups. Nobody else gave either of them a second glance, and once more it was an example of low-key inclusion in action. As another woman who uses the gym put it happily, 'we're coming out and being seen!'. Data such as these seem to challenge those aspects of social model writing about the body that appear to be based upon an extension of oppression theory, in assuming that disabled people are alienated from a general rush for bodily perfection (Stone, 1995). As these data suggest, both disabled and non-disabled people at Greenways seemed to be just as interested in using the venue as a social outlet as they were in improving their fitness levels and body shape. Thus it may be too simplistic to assume that all non-disabled people have bought into the myth of the perfect body (Hughes and Paterson, 1997; Paterson and Hughes, 1999; Stone, 1995), and that the drive towards bodily perfection at all costs is endemic in all leisure centres. Further, the data on individual disabled people's participation in Centre activities suggest that leisure settings like this one can provide spaces for disabled people to celebrate their impaired and sporting bodies as acts of resistance against mainstream assumptions of impairment as unmitigated personal tragedy, and of impaired bodies as being ugly or unacceptable. Such acts also challenge the implicit value judgement contained in Wolfensberger's concept of the 'conservatism corollary' (1992), which suggests that disabled people should do all they can to fit in with the mainstream, and avoid doing anything that would bring attention to their difference. Far from it – at Greenways at least some disabled people were 'out' and proud of it. Thus leisure participation seems to offer opportunities in parallel with the disability arts movement for impaired bodies to be celebrated as an integral part of individual identity, and as a cause for joy rather than sorrow (Swain and French, 2000). In that respect, participation in sport and leisure can be seen more as another expression of emancipatory politics than as a frantic attempt to deny the reality of impairment through an obsession with the body project.

However, it would be a mistake to claim that all disabled people who used the Centre were able to control their own impression management or to express themselves in such positive ways. For example, it was noticeable that, in contrast to individual users and the high-achieving Special Olympics groups, very few of the disabled people who visited as part of other segregated activity groups were given the opportunity to change into sports clothing before taking part, instead retaining their normal outdoor clothes throughout. Support staff told me that this was because they did not have time to help group members get changed into sports gear. However, the effects of this administrative decision on the participants, and on their potential to enjoy ordinary interactions with other Centre users, appeared to be wholly negative. Indeed, it was a good example of what Wolfensberger (1992: 45) meant when he said that services for disabled people are often designed with the needs of the service providers and funders in mind, rather than those of the service users. In this case, the negative effects on the participants of having to keep their outdoor clothing on were as follows. First, it served to make them stand out even more clearly from everyone else, and to brand them openly as 'Other' in a way that was devaluing (Race, 1999: 66; Wolfensberger, 1992: 41; Wolfensberger and Tullman, 1989: 213). Second, it suggested unconscious desires among the group leaders to keep impaired bodies – especially impaired bodies en masse – hidden from public view, in order to reduce the social anxiety which might otherwise arise in non-disabled people when confronted with 'unruly bodies and unruly minds' (Stanley and Wise, 1993: 197). Third, it implied that the group organizers did not see sports activities as providing an opportunity for the participants to take on socially valued roles that required the wearing of appropriate clothing. Instead, the sessions too often appeared to be viewed primarily as exercises in containment, designed to keep group members occupied in a secure setting for set periods of time.

Finally, group members who picked up on the negativity of these messages may as a result have seen no reason to push themselves to play an active sporting role, realizing that their efforts were unlikely to be rewarded. Certainly, in some segregated groups more than others, there was an over-whelming impression of apathy among the participants. Other possible reasons for this are discussed in subsequent chapters. For now, however, the main point to be made is that until group leisure centre visits by disabled people are properly staffed so that participants can change into sports clothes and start to feel the activity to be a real sporting event, many such sessions will continue to be at best mere exercises in containment, and at worst the active abuse of disabled people's identity and spirit.

Making connections through 'the communicative body'

Despite the necessarily negative tone of the conclusion to the last section, it was true that as an individual disabled person I found my own participation in sports activities at Greenways a truly empowering experience, as well as being a key to making connections with staff and customers. In trying to analyse what was going on here, I found Frank's concept of 'the communi-cative body' (1991: 79) particularly useful. Frank suggests that, for commu-nicative bodies, 'the body's contingency is no longer its problem but its possibility'. This is a concept with which I suspect many disabled people will empathize, being used to developing alternative strategies to counteract the limiting effects of some individual impairments. It is an adaptive state of mind and body which may also have further positive implications in terms of allowing for the possibility of making connections with other people through the mutual sharing of experience, and of learning more about oneself from such encounters. Or, as Frank puts it:

> the communicative body's desire is for dyadic expression, not monadic consumption. Whether it produces joy, sorrow, or anger, it uses itself to express these. This expression takes the form of dyadic sharing. In the further contingency of this sharing, the body has the potential for more diffuse realization.
>
> (ibid.: 80)

On the face of it, this is a profoundly optimistic assertion which points to the possibility of the development – through communication – of mutual under-standing between people from apparently different backgrounds and life experiences. However, it was necessary to test the theory against the reality of interactions at Greenways before reaching any firm conclusions. One way I did this was by seeing how far it could explain what was going on in my own interactions with James. Certainly, as I have discussed in previous chapters, when we first started working together we had problems understanding both where the other was coming from and what we expected from each other. Also, for myself, at the start of the research internalized oppression made it particularly difficult to deal with the differences between our bodies, especially given his much more athletic build. As a result I had to ask him not to watch me participate in any of the sports activities, because I felt so self-conscious. Actually he later revealed that he had got round this injunction by watching me from places where he knew I could not see him – which just goes to show that you can't trust anybody! But it did require a huge effort of will on my part not to run away the first time I actively knew he was there when I was working out. Still, in the event this proved to be a major transition point in the development of my self-esteem, in that once I was reassured that he had not run screaming from the sight of me, I was able to lose much of my former self-consciousness about my body image, and to enjoy more actively my participation. Additionally, I am sure that it was at least in part because of my bodily self-revelation, and his implicit understanding of how much it had taken for me to open myself up in that way, that he subsequently felt able to share with me some of his own experiences of discrimination. So this seems to give some validity to Frank's idea that our bodies are a key emotional outlet through which we can begin to make connections between our experiences.

Another way of testing for evidence of the communicative body at Greenways was, at interview, to ask members of staff about their experiences of working with disabled people, and to see how they reported those encounters. Specifically, I wanted to discover whether they always saw disabled people as 'Other', or as ordinary customers with whom they had been able to make connections. When questioned, most staff at first claimed that they had little experience of working with disabled people, but often as the interview progressed they would then proceed to casually tell me about times when they had worked with deaf people, or with people with learning difficulties, or people with any number of other impairments. Over time I realized that the apparent confusion here arose from their assumption that 'disabled people' always and only meant 'wheelchair users', a preconception that was no doubt fostered by my presence as a wheelchair-using researcher. As a result, I had to amend my interview protocol to include an explicit question about who came to mind when the phrase 'disabled person' was used, so that I could be sure we were talking about the same thing. In fact, the data collected confirmed my suspicion that most of them initially assumed that 'disabled person' equals 'wheelchair user'. This finding was confirmation of my belief that it may be necessary for disabled and non-disabled people to agree common meanings and associations for impairment-related terms before we can have meaningful discussions. Here, once we had discussed their assumptions and established a more holistic definition of 'disabled people', most were then forthcoming with information that suggested they were in practice often using social model principles of inclusion in their work, although none of them would have named it as such. For example, I routinely asked them whether they thought that working with disabled people required any special skills:

> A: I s'pose it's your own skills, and it's common sense, to a certain extent . . . common sense you wouldn't try to coach a deaf person and shout at them, 'cos that's not going to get you anywhere. But I don't think so – I think it's interpersonal skills, and just sort of common sense really, I'd say. So, I don't think you can have specific training on . . . it's like saying, 'well, if there's an irate customer you should handle them like this, but if there's a really friendly customer then you should handle them like this . . .' – now that's just common knowledge, isn't it? It's just like, if it's an irate customer you should try and calm them down, and reassure them, and if it's a really friendly customer then you're . . . really friendly back to them . . .

> B: The training aspect – I think it varies for every individual anyway, and I think you've got to be careful. I don't think people want treating any differently, most of the time. You've got to just – I think you get different things out of different people. You've got to treat them as a person, and individual, rather than a group anyway, even within the group.

> C: . . . I don't think that required any special skills, other than accepting people for what they are.

In general, then, there was resistance to any idea that leisure staff would always need extra training before working with disabled people per se, because this seemed to them to imply wrongly that disabled people were automatically 'a problem'. However, some rightly pointed out the lack of training available to them even if they had wanted to specialize in working with disabled people. One instructor reported having to adapt her own son's physiotherapy exercises for use by the disability groups to whom she taught aerobics, because there was no specialist adaptive training available. Others, too, highlighted the current lack of training courses on offer which would give mainstream leisure instructors the additional skills they wanted in order to help them to make more of their sessions inclusive. Yet since the fieldwork ended I have discovered from sources outside the Centre that training courses in leisure provision are available for social services staff who work exclusively with disabled people. However, Greenways staff were seemingly unaware of such training opportunities. This suggests the presence of an unnecessary structural barrier, in which only social services staff, seen as accredited disability professionals, are offered training which might actually be equally – perhaps even more – appropriate for staff from leisure organizations. It also suggests the ongoing segregation of provision for disabled people from ordinary mainstream activities, if only those participating in segregated social service-led sessions can benefit from such expertise. As such, the lack of more widely available training represents yet another structural barrier to inclusion.

In terms of general leisure provision, most staff at Greenways who I spoke to rejected any notion that existing mainstream intermediate and advanced level sessions should be slowed down and made easier to accommodate people with less experience or ability, since this would cause anger among those advanced users who had paid for more challenging courses. However, at least one instructor who held this view qualified it by saying that, where her own classes were too advanced for potential new recruits, she would give them information about other more appropriate sessions, even where this meant recommending courses at other Centres. This strategy would benefit less experienced disabled and non-disabled customers alike. Another advocated setting up a 'disabled club' at Greenways as a precursor to achieving full inclusion, explaining his reasoning thus:

> You know, one of the problems with the gym, particularly – non-disabled people or able-bodied people, they've got this image that a gym is full of beefcakes who do nothing but push weights, and they're like this kind of overweight, unfit, shrivelling kind of wreck, you know, and they just can't get over that barrier. They just think it's going to be so embarrassing and humiliating, and that's about able-bodied people, you know – so I would imagine it's like doubly bad for disabled people, 'cos they've got the, double the stigma. And I think if they had the opportunity to come in and use it as a group, that would be a fantastic opportunity for them then to get the kind of confidence and skills that they need, and then to come in whenever they wanted . . . I think one of the spin-offs of that would be that actually staff would get used to dealing with people with disabilities, and therefore when they are in an inclusive environment then ordinary people can see the staff totally confident in dealing with disabled people, and the whole thing will rub off, and it will become a normal activity.

To me, this response shows 'the communicative body' in action, demonstrating how the physical and coaching interplay between individuals has the potential to teach each of them about the other so that eventually the fear of difference vanishes and inclusion is achieved. At a more pragmatic level, the principle discussed here of disabled people using segregated sessions as confidence-building staging posts on the route to inclusion has already been used successfully in other recreation settings (BT/The Fieldfare Trust, 1997). However, it was only suggested on this one occasion by a member of staff at Greenways who was also – and probably not by coincidence – the parent of a disabled child. That others did not discuss the possibility of moving from segregated to inclusive provision perhaps resulted from the structural barrier that all the segregated group sessions were run by external contract staff, so that segregation in that setting became something of a self-fulfilling prophecy. In other words, to staff with limited experience of working with disabled people it perhaps appeared that anyone who needed to join a segregated group must have such complex support needs that they could only ever be catered for in such specialist groups. And yet, in their casual interactions with group members whom they met around the Centre, Greenways staff actually often displayed more inclusive behaviour than did the so-called disability professionals. It was unfortunate that during the fieldwork staffing and funding shortages made it impossible for Greenways staff to implement my suggestion that they might become involved in the running of some of the segregated sessions, since that would have been a highly practical way both of breaking down some of the existing structural barriers in those groups, and of increasing Greenways staff's expertise in working with disabled people. Nevertheless, the extracts used in this section reflected a willingness by Centre staff to treat disabled people as ordinary customers. As they became increasingly conscious over time of the new organizational imperatives to reduce the Centre's debt and to generate new income, they appeared to become even more open to the possibilities offered by disabled people as a new and as yet relatively untapped source of revenue. Realistically, it is perhaps only when the economic advantages of inclusive practice are pointed out to organizations in this way that they will become fully committed to improving both physical and programme access.

Some conclusions

The Greenways data suggest that in this ex-local authority setting many users were more concerned with issues of body maintenance and the prevention of further deterioration than with narcissistic attempts to cultivate the body beautiful (Giddens, 1991). In this setting, too, individual people with impairments were free to join in, with that participation being the key to inclusion, regardless of actual physical ability. Many of those individuals, myself included, clearly enjoyed being ordinary players, and some overtly expressed their satisfaction at disrupting mainstream assumptions about the need to keep impaired bodies hidden through their active participation in activities alongside non-disabled people. Such acts of resistance are due cause for celebration. As the data show, however, not all disabled people who used the Centre had the opportunity to express their embodiment like this, being forced to keep their bodies hidden due to structural barriers expressed as 'staff shortages'. The interviews with Centre staff uncovered

other, related, structural barriers that appear – in the light of evidence uncovered since the fieldwork finished – to show a preference within the
social services system to keep their professional knowledge to themselves
rather than sharing it with teachers and coaches from other professions.
Unsurprisingly, it is disabled people who may be expected to lose most
from the maintenance of such barriers.

To end on a more positive note, however, this chapter has also discussed
the applicability of elements of Frank's concept of 'the communicative
body' to my observation of disabled/non-disabled interactions at Greenways. I would want to interview more disabled people about their experiences before making any generalized conclusions, but certainly I found
Frank's analysis useful in explaining the symbiotic nature of many of my
own relationships with staff and customers at Greenways, and I know it is
one which I could equally apply to many of my relationships in other
settings. Having said that, the example I have given here of the initial difficulty I found in expressing my own relative physical vulnerability in front
of James is also instructive. As a result of this experience, I am extremely
conscious that it is no 'small ask' to be suggesting to other disabled people
that adopting a strategy of self-revelation with non-disabled people may be
a necessary step towards breaking down assumptions of a binary opposition
between us. An essential proviso to such a strategy is that there will always
be occasions when such tactics will be too dangerous and the need for self-
protection must prevail instead. Nor am I advocating an approach in
which, as too often previously, disabled people have been expected to
reveal all while their non-disabled interrogators reveal nothing of themselves. Rather, to work in the manner that Frank suggests, the self-revelation
has to come from both parties.

Perhaps this suggestion borders on the naive, in assuming that existing
power relations can be overcome in this way. However, at an individual
level it has sometimes worked for me, and may have the potential for
wider application, although some cultural barriers may need to be overcome
in the process. For example, one of my non-disabled friends, with whom
I have a lot in common in terms of background and life experience, was
initially reticent about claiming that her experience was similar to mine,
because she felt that I must automatically have had a much harder life
than her because of my status as a disabled person. However, as bell hooks
has said of her experience within one ethnically mixed women's group:

> We talked about the need to acknowledge that we all suffer in some way,
> but that we are not all oppressed or equally oppressed. Many of us
> feared that our experiences were irrelevant because they were not as
> oppressive or as exploited as the experiences of others. We discovered
> that we had a greater feeling of unity when people focused truthfully

on their own experiences without comparing them with those of others in a competitive way.

(2000: 59)

For my friend and myself, it was only through learning to acknowledge that each of our sets of experience was valid, albeit sometimes in different ways, that we were able to break through the cultural barrier which had originally made her assume that our differences were always more important than our commonality. I suggest that such adaptive strategies may be essential in the future if Finkelstein's call (1996: 11) for disabled people to form alliances with other groups in the struggle to achieve change is to be implemented effectively. In short, I believe that disabled and non-disabled people may need to learn to trust each other enough to be able to share something of our views and experiences, and to recognize that each person's perspective is valid in its own right, if future cross-group alliances are to become sufficiently cohesive to bring about social change.

This chapter has addressed some issues around disabled people's embodiment, and has suggested benefits which may be gained both from embracing the fact of that embodiment, and from in turn using it as a means of uncovering limited areas of commonality with the experiences of non-disabled people through the 'communicative body' (Frank, 1991). In the next chapter, by way of contrast, I look at some situations at Greenways where no such positive connections between disabled and non-disabled people were in evidence, and where instead disabled people were on the receiving end of disablist oppression.

Chapter II

Being a disabled person

General examples of disabling language and actions

As I mentioned in Chapter 4, throughout the fieldwork I was careful not to challenge the use of inappropriate disabling terminology by non-disabled people at Greenways, because I wanted the data to reflect their current constructions of disability. I was also concerned that if I started off by questioning their use of language they might become so guarded in what they said to me that my opportunities for further data collection would become limited. This acceptance strategy appeared to work, in that it showed up the ongoing use of inappropriate and oppressive language to describe disabled customers of the leisure centre. Among the most frequently used inappropriate terms were 'confined to a wheelchair' and 'the mentally handicapped', although I sometimes noticed people would hastily correct themselves to use other, less judgemental, phrases such as 'wheelchair user' or 'people with learning difficulties' when they saw that I was within earshot. On the positive side, this showed that at least people did make the effort to change their language when I was around. However, the experience also suggested that they were not fully committed to using appropriate terminology consistently when they could still get away with using outdated terms when speaking to other non-disabled people. Staff reactions to Vicky, described in Chapter 6, also supported my suspicions that sometimes there was an associated infantilization of disabled people in the way in which they were spoken to and described, or else an assumption was made that their efforts – however commendable – would never quite be up to the mark. For example, I overheard one activity group leader being referred to in patronizing terms by his non-disabled volunteers as 'the wheelchair lad', and in my own case my support worker was told by an activity leader that, 'of course, Claire tries her best, but she's very limited . . .'. Interestingly, both of these comments were made by non-Greenways staff, and I can think of few occasions over the seven months when an in-house member of staff made an inappropriate disabling comment about disabled customers direct to my face. Taken as a whole, the findings reported here do however suggest that initiatives aimed at developing a common language with which disabled and non-disabled people can discuss issues around disability and impairment may meet with resistance, or be treated with lip-service by some non-disabled people.

During the interviews with the staff I also noticed a strong demarcation between the ways in which they described wheelchair users compared with other disabled people. In that recreation setting, wheelchair users were always defined as 'disabled', whereas all other people with impairments were described as 'normal' or 'nearly normal'. It was clear, then, that being able to walk was seen as a major indicator of people's ability to take part in sport. At the same time, however, most staff showed little understanding of access issues or 'impairment effects' (Thomas, 1999) that might have a negative impact on ambulant disabled people's ability to participate in Centre activities. This was unfortunate, since my observation of the layout and management of Greenways suggested several ways in which programme access for this much larger group of disabled people could have been improved. These included producing information about the Centre's leisure activities in alternative formats (for example, in large print, on tape, and taped in other community languages) to reach a wider market audience; ensuring that the whole of the venue was well-lit and that directional signage used good colour contrasts so that people with visual impairments could find their way around the site independently; installing hearing induction loops at reception points and in teaching areas, and reducing the use of background music in sessions attended by people with hearing impairments, so that they would be more likely to pick up on what the session leader was saying; providing session leaders with disability equality training to increase their awareness of disabled people's needs; and offering discounted entry prices for disabled people and any essential support workers.

A clear starting point for such an improvements programme would be the provision of disability equality training, to give staff the knowledge they clearly need so that they can tailor their service provision to meet the needs of all disabled people. Having said that, the picture at Greenways was not one of completely exclusionary behaviour. At interview some staff were able to relate our discussion of disabling barriers to their own experience of having family members with illnesses and impairments, or of access problems they themselves had encountered when out in public places with children or grandchildren in pushchairs. This comparison was often made as a first step towards acknowledging wider links between disabled and non-disabled people's experience. My observation of coaching practice also showed that staff with no prior experience of working with disabled people, but who had a clear commitment to customer service, had recognized the need to adapt their service provision to meet disabled people's individual requirements. The key factor here seemed to be that of people's professional pride in wanting to deliver a good service, and about having the imagination to adapt their programmes where necessary (or indeed, to recommend a more appropriate alternative course or facility), to meet the needs of their customers.

Situational disablism

At an individual level, as time went on I became aware of the existence of situational disablism at the site, by which I mean that some people reacted to me in different ways according to who else happened to be around at the time. Two examples spring to mind here, one involving a member of the Centre's staff, and the other an external contractor. First, one day a young woman lifeguard was assigned to help me make notes while I was carrying out an access audit of part of the site. While we were working together she was extremely helpful, and even made one or two suggestions herself about features that seemed to need adapting. I felt that we had got on well together, and was looking forward to speaking to her again. However, the next few times I saw her she was with the male lifeguards, and on each of these occasions she completely ignored me. It felt as if she was embarrassed to be seen to acknowledge me when she was with her male friends, an impression which was compounded when by contrast I saw her on her own, or with other women, when she did always smile and say hello. I don't think it was pure disablism at work here. The fact that she only ignored me when she was with men suggested that gender forces and conditioning were affecting the encounter as well, and that as a very young woman she may have felt social pressures to present the body beautiful (untainted by contact with the likes of me), in ways which the older female members of staff were more able to resist. Still, whatever her motivation for acting as she did, the result was to make me feel hurt and excluded.

The second example came from my interactions with a local council worker. Again, the first time we met she acted in an inclusive way, and we had a serious discussion about aspects of my research, including the possibility of my being given access to the council's statistics on community use of leisure facilities. However, the second time we met was during a junior wheelchair basketball event at the Centre, which was attended by the mayor and other civic dignitaries. In fact, I only discovered when I arrived to observe proceedings that, although it was called a 'wheelchair basketball tournament', it was really a glorified simulation exercise designed to allow non-disabled children to try out playing basketball using wheelchairs. As I share the disability movement's disapproval of the use of simulation exercises like these for training purposes, I realized from the start that I was in a situation where I was likely to feel uncomfortable. Therefore initially I was pleased to see a familiar face in the form of this council worker. However, on this occasion she behaved in a completely different way towards me. First she came over, invaded my personal space by leaning in an overfamiliar way on the handles of my chair, and then suggested that I should 'have a go' and take part in the tournament. This was insulting on two grounds. For one thing, I was twenty years older than the participants, which I guess she thought didn't matter because it was after all 'only' wheelchair sport. Further, with my level of impairment there was no way I could have joined in even if I had wanted to. Rather than create a scene and jeopardize the future of the research, I just said 'no, I have enough trouble playing hockey', and left it at that. Shortly afterwards I heard her say in a cosy tone to one of the other officials 'I told her she should have a go, but she wouldn't'. It seemed, then, that among a group of predominantly non-disabled people bent on doing good she couldn't behave normally with me, but had to be seen to be following the role of paternalistic encourager of (supposedly) weak disabled people. I felt dreadful afterwards that I had not taken a stand and confronted her about her behaviour, regardless of the effect such action might have had on my research. Instead, I managed to internalize the oppression until the whole incident felt like my fault. This was one occasion where I would definitely have benefited from the presence of other disabled people as allies at the site, because it was simply too much for me to challenge the situation on my own. Again, then, the result of a non-disabled person's actions was to make me feel excluded and worthless.

Treatment of segregated disability group customers

From a research point of view, one of the advantages of my impairment is that I can easily pass as a person with learning difficulties. During the fieldwork I took advantage of this to participate in several segregated group activities at the Centre run primarily for people with learning difficulties, in order to compare the level of service they received with that which I experienced as an individual Centre user. With the proviso that most of those groups had to use segregated access routes to get to their activities, and were not given the opportunity to change into sports clothes, some of this segregated provision was otherwise appropriate and respectful of the participants, especially a group which was run by a member of the local council's community recreation team. He led by example in treating people as ordinary, and the atmosphere within that group was vibrant and happening, with people being out to have a good (and noisy) time. Once I saw him casually sit down in someone's vacant wheelchair to do some paperwork, and the fact that he did this perfectly naturally and without apparent forethought suggested that he did not see impairment-related equipment as devalued or to be avoided at all costs for fear of contamination. I suspect that his inclusive approach may have been partly due to his own experience of coming from a mixed-race background, which might in turn have made him more aware of equality issues and of the need to treat people as ordinary participants. Additionally, his background as a recreation professional may be relevant here, in that his primary role was to enable people to participate in recreation activities. This contrasted with the self-reported remit of some social services staff working with groups at the site, which was to keep those disabled people under surveillance. My view as to why this difference in approach existed is based on my observations both during this fieldwork and during my previous work as a recreation professional, which had shown up similar anomalies. These experiences suggest to me that how people react around each other is in part conditioned by their purpose in coming together. Thus it appeared that leisure staff and disabled people were routinely able to work together on an equitable basis because the main reason for them coming together was a factor external but common to each party – namely, a shared desire to participate in and enjoy leisure activities. Too often, however, when social services staff and disabled people came together at Greenways, it was on the basis of the supposed deficit of disabled people and the supposed technical expertise of the disability professionals. Neither side seemed able to break out of this professional–incompetent binary on which their relationship in other settings was based, to focus on the common goal here of enjoying their participation in leisure.

For much of the fieldwork this contrasting approach to service provision was evident. By and large, the groups run by recreation professionals appeared to facilitate disabled people's active participation in sport, whereas those run by social services staff seemed aimed primarily at containment and keeping disabled people sedentary and quiet for the duration of their visit. As one person from social services put it, 'We have to keep them all in one place, you know'. Yet this containment approach, combined with other aspects of service provision such as the failure to enable disabled people to change into sports clothes discussed in the previous chapter, appears to be inconsistent with normalization/SRV principles. It is hard to see how such segregative actions are compatible with the normalization/SRV aim of supporting disabled people to acquire and practise competencies that will improve their social image and enable them to take on successfully community-based socially valued roles (Wolfensberger, 1992: 34). Yet many of the practices witnessed during this research seemed more likely to reinforce negative responses to disabled people's difference, than to facilitate their social inclusion (ibid.: 42). This suggests that the disability staff concerned were either unaware of normalization/SRV principles, or else they failed to recognize that this leisure setting represented an appropriate venue in which they could be applied. However, as the White Paper *Valuing People* makes clear:

> Enabling people to use a wider range of leisure opportunities can make a significant contribution to improving quality of life, can help to tackle social exclusion, and encourage healthy lifestyles.
>
> (Department of Health, 2001: 80)

Thus disability service providers need to acknowledge that improving access to leisure for disabled people is now on the government's agenda, and that they may be expected to include leisure in individual and community care plans in the future (ibid.: 80). In turn this will require the provision of leisure opportunities that facilitate inclusion rather than reinforcing the devaluing of disabled people.

The growing impression gained during the research of disabled people being devalued by some disability services staff became more marked as a result of the time I spent with one particular social services-run group, which met weekly at the Centre. For several weeks after I first started working at Greenways I had heard Centre staff talking about this particular group, usually in glowing terms. I was told, for example, that 'they more or less have the run of the place', and that 'they do what they want'. The more I heard, the more impressed I was that a group of disabled people seemed so fully included in the life of the place. Expecting a group of hard-playing 'super-crips' (Morris, 1991), I became rather nervous about meeting them, in case my own sporting performance fell too far short of their standards. However, as I was to discover, the hype was somewhat at odds with the reality, as this extract from my field notes shows:

> I am thrust into the room and left to it by Jane, who says 'This is Claire, who I told you about', and then leaves immediately. In the somewhat dim light I thread my way past the backs of two other wheelchair users, and find a gap in the group circle. Most of the staff are smoking. One is reading the paper, apparently trying to put off the moment where interaction with the others is inevitable. None of the other disabled people present meets my eye, or displays any outward sign of awareness that I am there. I recognize and respect this strategy . . . A female member of staff turns to me and starts asking me about my chair. Inevitably this leads on to a discussion of 'other wheelchair users/people with cp I have known'. I pretend interest, and at the same time wonder if she realizes that looking at a point around the middle of my forehead does not really count as eye contact . . . Next I watch as the group leader, acting out 'Paternalistic Facilitator', puts his arm along the back of the seat and leans towards the new group member, a woman whom someone has already told me has a progressive impairment, as he seemingly explains to her how the group operates. As I watch I wonder if she's realized yet how casually exposed membership of such a group may make her. And I know that segregated facilities have their place, but sometimes privacy is so hard to maintain as a result . . . A short diversion is caused by the late arrival of another group member, together with a young male support worker. In the latter I suspect a junior version of the group leader, and am not disappointed, as he proceeds to strut his stuff in front of his audience.

I tune out of listening to what he's saying in order to watch the game going on in front of me, but can't help wondering why it is necessary for some support workers to talk so loudly at people. Are they afraid nobody will take enough notice of them if they don't?

From my observation, far from being an all-action group of sporting supremos, apart from one short morning activity session this group seemed to spend most of their all-day visits to Greenways sitting in one room while the staff smoked, read the paper, and swapped unfunny jokes. For the most part the staff appeared oblivious to their presence, and did nothing to alleviate the increasing distress of some group members resulting from this inactivity and lack of stimulation. Being stuck in a stuffy smoky room with this staff menagerie felt to me like being in the inner circle of hell – and I knew that I was free to leave at any time. I hate to think what effect long-term exposure to such oppression was having on the regular group members. It was staff behaviour of a type which I had previously only observed in the worst of residential centres, and which they appeared to have imported wholesale into this recreation setting. The strength of such stereotyped roles was such that they made absolutely no attempt to modify their behaviour when I or members of the Centre staff were around. It seemed indeed that they felt totally secure in their unquestioned authority over the disabled people in their 'care'. My first encounter with this group left me stunned, unable to believe that behaviour like this was tolerated at an otherwise inclusive setting. My second (I was only able to cope with two such meetings) confirmed my earlier suspicions of inappropriate behaviour, and left me furious. It was at this point that I took action by reporting the group leader to James, the consequences of which are described in Chapter 13.

In trying to make sense of why the group leader and some of his staff acted in such routinely oppressive ways towards the people they were meant to be supporting, I felt that explanations at several different levels were possible. At its most basic, this was a stark example of the way that some non-disabled people use their situational power over disabled people to further oppress them. I found this situation completely intolerable, and the bottom line was that I had to report their actions to James. However, I was also aware that there may have been deeper reasons behind their actions. This does not in any way justify what they were doing, but may suggest the need to review some aspects of community care provision. In particular, Smith and Brown (1992) have identified the lack of support for community-based disability staff as being one of the major shortcomings of the de-institutionalization process. They argue that the old mental handicap institutions served a containment function for such staff, which protected them from internalizing the stress associated with care work; and suggest that what is missing from community care is 'a repository for collective projections of madness and difference; and an organizational structure that contain the anxiety aroused by caring for people perceived to be "different"' (ibid.: 88). In the absence of proper organizational support to manage this distress, staff may be forced to develop their own coping strategies. Thus, at a psychological level, the need expressed by disability staff at Greenways to keep the group in one place and under surveillance at all times could have been related to their dislike of the 'burden of care'. As Obholzer and Zagier Roberts explain:

> To be 'weighed down by responsibility' invites flight from the caring task, which can at times be hateful. Obsessional routines of care can serve to protect patients from carers' unconscious hate, from what staff fear they might do to those in their charge if not controlled by rigid discipline.
>
> (1994: 83)

A similar case is made by Sinason:

> Being close to something that has gone wrong is a permanent reminder of the frailty of the human body and mind. Where staff are not helped to deal with that there is no possibility of an attempt to link the incontinence to any emotional disturbance or to anger or depression. There is no attempt to think of a behavioural programme or provide such facilities as art or music or drama therapy.
>
> (1992: 208)

Other related psychological reasons may help to further explain the practical failure of this set of staff to provide appropriate and fulfilling activities for the people they were working with, as Conboy-Hill suggests:

> It might be argued . . . that denial of emotional functioning in disabled people has been a central factor in our ability to see as satisfactory the sorts of life-styles such people have been required to live. In other words, failure to recognize the impact of loss on people with learning disability arises directly from our need to see such people as lacking in effective emotional apparatus, thereby justifying unacceptably barren life-styles. This conveniently feeds into our own need to avoid discussion of pain and grief and so the cycle of ignorance and inaction has been perpetuated.
>
> (1992: 151)

The interconnections between the effects of de-institutionalization and the application of normalization/SRV principles in community-based care may also be relevant here. Brown (1992: 188) has commented that one of the problems with normalization/SRV approaches is that the staff who are expected to deliver these programmes are taught about the concept '*as if it were something outside of themselves*'. In other words, these inadequately supported community staff are not encouraged to see any similarity between their clients' experiences and their own. In particular, they are not asked to make connections by recognizing the ways in which they themselves have previously had to try to make sense of their own differences from ideals of behaviour and performance in making their way in the world, in the way that they are now encouraging the disabled people they work with to do. Seeing this personal growth process as being somehow different for people with learning difficulties may then make it harder for these staff to support them properly as they too work towards making sense of their differences from the ideal.

These explanations make a lot of sense to me. However, I will never know for sure if some of the staff working with that group were weighed down by the burden of care, or would ever consciously concede that they either hated the disabled people they worked with or saw them as in some way less than human, for the simple reason that I never felt strong enough to confront them about their behaviour. Even when I met them in the group setting they had the power to silence me within minutes through their words, behaviour and the unspoken assumptions about who was in charge that permeated all of our exchanges. I knew that I would never be able to take on the task of interviewing them one to one as well, because their oppression of me was too strong. As a result, this was probably the most significant occasion during the research when I would have benefited from working in partnership with a non-disabled researcher, since they would have been able to conduct such an interview at less personal risk, and might have been able to confirm why this particular group of staff worked in such oppressive ways.

Stereotyping of disabled people and its effects

As the research progressed, I discovered that it was not only the disability professionals who believed that disabled people needed special separate leisure services. Given the apparently high level of awareness among Centre staff of the persistence of disabling barriers, and their inclusive approach with individual disabled customers, it came as a surprise to find that some of them seemed at the same time to hold negative and stereotyped views of those disabled customers who visited the Centre as part of segregated groups. Further, it appeared that these attitude barriers were being used to justify ongoing differential service provision for those groups. For example, when I asked why he thought most members of those groups tended not to mix with other Centre users, but socialized in a separate room instead, one person gave a range of individualized reasons which were fairly typical of the responses I received:

> I think it's probably because they can manoeuvre their wheelchairs better . . . Some of them are able to manage on their own, but some of them have to have their carers with them. They can't really manage on their own . . . they probably find it a little bit more private up here . . . if they're having little meetings – particularly the carers – then they can keep their eye on them better here . . .

A number of issues are raised in this short extract. First, there was an assumption that space was an issue for the group users. It undoubtedly was, but the implication here was that organizing separately as a result was an appropriate solution, rather than removing structural access barriers to inclusion at other points around the site. Second, this is another example of the infantilization of disabled people, in the assumption that group members always needed support, and that they would only ever have 'little meetings', not full-blown serious ones. Finally, and chillingly, the supposed need for surveillance of disabled people by disability service staff is once again stated unquestioningly.

For a while I wrestled with the apparent contradiction here, that Centre staff who behaved in generally inclusive ways with me and other individual disabled people seemed to revert to stereotyped disabling views when discussing members of segregated groups. Eventually, however, I surmised that one reason for such oppressive practice was their apparent unease at the size of these groups. In other words, they were able to cope perfectly well in interactions with individual disabled people, but were fazed by the appearance of disabled people en masse. Such a reaction would not be without precedent, given that a similar process occurred during the transition from a feudal to a capitalist society in Britain. Whereas previously one or two disabled people might have lived in each small community, and been more or less accepted within it, now suddenly there were large numbers of disabled people in the new conurbations (Finkelstein, 1980). I believe that the administrative response of incarceration was not entirely about separating off those who could no longer contribute their labour to the new means of production (Oliver, 1996), but was also at least partly born out of non-disabled people's fear of being swamped by all these disabled people who appeared to threaten the new capitalist normative standards of productivity. Certainly, as Scull has pointed out (1993: 82), some of the asylums built during the early nineteenth century were bigger than the factories of the time, which may have added to a psychological impression that suddenly there were overwhelming numbers of disabled people within society. At a time of social upheaval and displacement from the old certainties of rural life in small and stable communities, anyone who looked or acted differently may have seemed to pose a threat to non-disabled people who were themselves desperately seeking new roles and stability in the developing industrial age. Perhaps, then, it was not surprising that the reaction was to shut away all those disabled people who showed that actually not everyone could be forced to adapt to the newly regulated ways of working and living. 'Out of sight, out of mind' may thus have been a psychological as well as an administrative response (Brown and Smith, 1992).

Nowadays, a policy of decarceration and community care may mean that more disabled people live in the outside world. However, it seems that older associations of fear and of being overwhelmed by large numbers of people who challenge society's perception of 'normality' persist, and still have the power to affect non-disabled people's responses to impairment. This was shown a few years ago when a group of deaf people was asked to leave a holiday camp because they were alleged to be disturbing other holiday-makers by their use of sign language (Anon: 1998). It might be argued that actually it was less their use of signing than the fact that there were a lot of them doing it which subconsciously posed a threat to the oral culture. One person doing something different could be explained away as an aberration, whereas a whole group of people behaving differently might actively threaten the status quo.

If fear of large groups of disabled people is indeed an issue for non-disabled people, it is perhaps not surprising that Greenways staff resorted to stereotyping when faced – as was often the case – with group visits by forty to fifty disabled people. As Gilman has explained:

> Stereotypes can and often do exist parallel to the ability to create sophis-ticated rational categories that transcend the crude line of difference present in the stereotype. We retain our ability to distinguish the 'indi-vidual' from the stereotyped class into which the object might auto-matically be placed . . . for the non-pathological individual the stereotype is a momentary coping mechanism, one that can be used and then discarded once anxiety is overcome.
>
> (1997: 285)

Unfortunately, because the policy of mass group provision persisted rather than also encouraging small group or individual visits, many of the Centre staff never seemed able to get past seeing those group members in stereo-typed terms in the same way as they could in their interactions with indi-vidual disabled people. Nor was the situation helped by the practice of staffing the groups with external contractors rather than with Greenways staff, a barrier which only served to perpetuate the 'them and us' atmo-sphere. These findings therefore support the normalization/SRV approach that disabled people may be best supported to participate in community-based activities as individuals or in very small groups (Wolfensberger, 1992). Having to participate in large groups alongside forty or fifty other people is, after all, hardly conducive to anyone being able to meet and socialize with people outside that group. At Greenways this approach served merely to reinforce a sort of siege mentality within the groups, with the members being herded in and out of the building en masse, while the disability staff shouted at anyone they felt wasn't moving fast enough or who was 'drawing attention to themselves' by their appearance or behaviour. Quite apart from the low-quality leisure experience for the group members that resulted from this dehumanizing treatment, none of this was likely to help non-disabled people at the site move beyond false stereotyped views of people with learning difficulties as unruly, dangerous and not worth getting to know.

Demarcation through disabling practices

In addition to the disablist oppression caused by the policy of mass group leisure provision, and the ways that practices such as making people wear their outdoor clothing while playing sport acted as a means of demarcation between groups of disabled people and other Centre users, and between the groups and their staff, I also uncovered other examples of disabling practices. For example, on more than one occasion I saw Susan, a wheelchair user, arriving for her session being pushed along by a council transport driver. Even in hot weather, when the drivers were wearing shorts and t-shirts, I noticed that they also wore heavy-duty industrial gloves while they were pushing her chair. The first time I saw this I assumed that the driver concerned had a skin complaint that meant that he had to keep his hands covered. However, as soon as he had left Susan I saw him pull the gloves off in evident relief. At this point I realized that he had only been wearing them so that he did not have to come into skin contact with her chair. It was as if she was seen as a piece of hazardous waste to be dealt with, and it made me feel sick to the core. I just hoped that because he was standing behind her she had not seen what he had done. Subsequently I watched her arrival on several other occasions and each time, whoever the driver was, the same performance took place, which raises the question of whether it might be council policy for their transport workers to wear heavy-duty gloves when handling disabled people. If so, it needs to be changed, since it sends such wholly inappropriate messages both to disabled people and anyone else who happens to witness it about disabled people being, literally, untouchable.

Sometimes non-disabled people appeared to be so scared of disabled people that they avoided them altogether. Once I observed a couple come out of the gym and head straight into the bar for a drink, only to reappear within seconds, looking uncomfortable. One reason for this may have been that a group of disabled people were already in there. I was also told that even some of the Centre staff would walk the long way around the building in order not to have to come into contact with the disability groups. Equally, as James and others made clear towards the end of my research, not everyone had been comfortable about my own presence at the site. For example, I was told that some members of staff had avoided talking to me for the entire seven months because they were afraid that they would not be able to understand my speech. In similar vein, the site manager only formally introduced himself to me after I had been there for three months, and then was at pains to tell me how relaxed he was around disabled people because he had a disabled relative. Unfortunately, past experience has suggested to me that often the people who go out of their way to explain how much they know about disabled people are in reality those least at ease with the situation. Sometimes it feels as if they make such statements in an effort to reassure themselves that they truly can cope. Certainly it does little to reassure me. It is often far easier to deal with people who make no such claims to 'expert knowledge', but who simply act in an ordinary inclusive manner.

Another factor which seemed to affect Centre staff's attitudes was an apparent perception that the disability professionals who worked with the groups must know what they were doing, and be acting in the best interests of the group members. In a way this finding should not have surprised me, since leisure managers usually trust the teachers and youth workers who use their facilities to manage their groups appropriately. However, in the case of the segregated disability groups this laissez-faire approach had unfortunate consequences in terms of the way that some disabled people were treated. Hence, as discussed earlier, Centre staff accepted the apparent need for the surveillance of group members simply because the group's staff had told them it was necessary. Further, they actually seemed unable to challenge such views even where they themselves had misgivings about some of the things they saw going on. For example, when I reported to James my experience of inappropriate behaviour in the segregated group described above, I found that as soon as I opened the conversation he came out with a whole series of points of his own about the way the group was being run, many of which mirrored my own unspoken concerns. What I found worrying, however, was the fact that although he had clearly been concerned about the group for some time, he needed me (as a supposed expert in the field) to raise the issue first, and had been unable to tackle the situation independently without my confirmation that his instinct was correct. This incident points to the extreme power which disability professionals have to control medicalized disability discourse, and the reluctance of non-disability professionals to challenge their authority. It also suggests a flaw in the normalization/SRV argument that community-based service provision should provide disabled people with additional safeguards against abuse because having other people around makes it more likely that they would step in and stop such abusive activity taking place (Race, 1999: 154). Instead, in this particular case the authority of the disability staff went unchallenged because the Centre staff assumed they must be acting appropriately. At its worst, such quiescence may be seen as part of a continuum of behaviour which ends in the mass murder of disabled people by eugenicists, because other people assume that the professionals must know what they are doing, and be acting for the common good. As such it is truly terrifying.

Some conclusions

This chapter has uncovered and discussed some examples of disabling practice at Greenways. In particular, it has focused on 'psycho-emotional' disabling barriers (Thomas, 1999), in the form of negative attitudes about disabled people, and the ways that psychological barriers were used by some disability staff to protect themselves from the stress of community-based care work. Although such barriers were harder to articulate and explain than the more obvious economic and physical access ones discussed in previous chapters, they were actually all the more dangerous as a result. As such they cannot be ignored, although overarching legislative solutions alone may be of little use because they allow for insufficiently individualized responses to particular instances of psychological oppression. Instead, alongside legislative change, specific remedies may be needed for each setting, together with a recognition at wider policy level of the need both to adequately support staff engaged in community-based support work, and to put in place adequate safeguards to more effectively protect against the abuse of disabled service users.

In my view, one practical way of tackling the disabling attitude barriers at Greenways would be, as previously suggested, for Centre staff to become more involved in the leadership and staffing of the segregated disability group activities. On the basis of my own experience of sporting participation at the site, I believe this would improve the range and quality of activities on offer to these groups. Such routine contact with disabled people would also in time enable Centre staff to see more of them as individuals rather than persisting with stereotyped views of devalued difference derived from some of the existing disability staff. Yet again, then, data in this chapter show the impossibility of understanding events at Greenways without taking account of the investments drawn from other professional environments that some participants brought into the setting. It shows the terrifying extent to which the dependency of disability professionals on disabled people (Oliver, 1990: 90–91) was obscured here by their oppression of the disabled people they were meant to be supporting, and supports the social model argument that the process of eradicating disability will depend on forcing change across multiple fields, or else a few 'bad apples' will be able to continue to exercise their power for evil in otherwise inclusive settings. In at least one case here, I could only see progress being made if the group leader was removed from post. While such individuals continue to control group provision, inclusion will never be achieved. Such research findings also lead me to question whether simply adopting normalization/SRV approaches could ever lead to disabled people's full inclusion in that setting. Although normalization/SRV aims to improve disability service provision, it stops short of challenging the wider power relations that give disability professionals more power and authority than disabled people (Oliver, 1996), arguing that attempting to change the power relations on which society is based is beyond its intended remit (Race, 1999; Wolfensberger, 1992). Yet as this chapter has shown, disability professionals do have power over disabled people, and not all of them use it in ways that support disabled people's social inclusion. Unless normalization/SRV programmes tackle this problem head on, it seems all too likely that disabled people will remain at risk of abuse.

Despite the specific problems with some of the group activities at Greenways, I believe that properly run segregated sessions can have a role in generating self-confidence and reducing disability among people with impairments. However, alongside this there is a definite need to look for ways of encouraging more informal interaction between those groups and other customers, by supporting disabled people to use the Centre at other times rather than always as part of the group, and introducing a subsidized pricing policy for mainstream activities in order to make this a practical option. In addition, more joint use of supposedly shared spaces like the café should be encouraged, rather than perpetuating the existing practice of group members eating food purchased at the café back in their separate room. This would however require the education of group leaders, and the removal of some access barriers such as the shortage of support staff.

In terms of educating Greenways staff, the provision of disability equality training would be valuable in further improving their service to customers. There was also some evidence that ongoing contact with me during the field-work enabled some people to move beyond their initial oppressive practice, as shown by the example given in Chapter 4 of the café worker who was much more friendly and helpful once she had got used to me being around. Also, towards the end of the project James told me that he had over-heard me being described as 'Claire, the woman doing the consultancy', rather than as 'Claire, the disabled person/wheelchair user', which suggested that I was increasingly being seen as a whole person instead of being identi-fied solely on the basis of my impairment status. What made this comment even more significant was that apparently the person who described me in this positive way had been one of those initially most concerned at the thought of me working there. Yet by the time I left I was told that my long-term presence around the Centre as a routine mainstream participant had helped many of the staff to see me as ordinary. These experiences suggest that employing more disabled people in the leisure industry would help speed up the inclusion process.

Having shown in this chapter some of the ways in which disabled people were oppressed at Greenways, in the next chapter I illustrate more of the complexities of power relations in that setting by revealing some of the ways in which my own practice oppressed other disabled people at the site.

Chapter 12

Being an oppressor

Using multiple identity as an excuse for oppression

As this book should have demonstrated by now, my understanding of both exclusionary and inclusive practice at Greenways was enhanced once I accepted that people were responding to me in different ways, and revealing different constructions of disability, according to which of my identities they saw as being primary at any one time. By ordering the data in terms of those identities, I have tried to show that in those various relationships I was not always a powerless victim, but instead occupied a range of positions, in some of which – such as recreation professional, consultant and friend – I too was able to exercise power. However, I was also aware that having power meant I was in danger of abusing it. In some of my dealings – especially those with other disabled people at the Centre – I know I didn't always get it right, and could be accused of oppressive practice.

The discussion of my oppressive practice that follows is based on two definitions. bell hooks sees oppression as 'the *absence of choices*' (2000: 5), while Vernon explains that:

> A fundamental dilemma rooted in oppression is that there are very few pure oppressors or pure victims. Even those who are themselves oppressed often consciously or unconsciously engage in the oppression of others who deviate from the established norm in a different way from them.
>
> (1999: 389)

Previously I have shown how my ability to pass as a person with learning difficulties helped me to conduct the research, and have described the ways in which a number of the people with learning difficulties I worked with showed me friendship and support. However, there were some occasions when I either consciously or unconsciously used my intelligence and my formal researcher role as distancing devices between us. Sometimes this was because I simply could not bear what I was seeing, as with the group discussed in the last chapter; while on other occasions I found that I was making assumptions about people's behaviour which were based on inappropriate normative values. In both situations, once I realized what I was doing I then had to make difficult personal decisions about whether and how to rectify my errors. This chapter will concentrate on discussing those situations where I chose to leave things as they were.

The bouncy castle episode

During my first observation session with one of the better-run segregated groups at Greenways, I noticed that some people were playing on a large bouncy castle. Later, during a conversation with one of the group leaders, he apologized to me for the presence of this piece of equipment, saying that he was aware that a bouncy castle was not an age-appropriate activity for adults, but that it had been introduced as a temporary measure while the trampoline which they normally used during the session was being repaired. At the time I accepted this explanation because I agreed that the bouncy castle wasn't age-appropriate equipment for an adult-only group, and over the course of the next few months I kept my eye on the situation to see when the castle would once again be replaced by the trampoline. However, this didn't happen, and so towards the end of the fieldwork I was preparing to include the scenario in my research report as another example of the infantilization of disabled people at the site.

Then, during my last session with the group, one of the members came up to me with a petition she wanted me to sign. She had organized this in response to the staff's intention, as previously reported to me, to remove the bouncy castle and reinstate the trampoline. In seeking to challenge this decision, her view was that actually the group members wanted to have a choice between using either piece of equipment, and that as a result both should be on offer all the time. Then she said:

> The staff don't like the bouncy castle because they say it's not age-appropriate. But some of the people who come to this group need to go back before they can go forward, and the castle helps them to do that.

This statement was full of insight, and mirrored almost exactly what Sinason has said about her own experience of using psychotherapy with people with learning difficulties:

> Having the power to make something else make a sound or move can help some patients express their feelings about their own inability to control these activities in their own bodies. Some of my colleagues who work only with adults have been concerned that 'toys' might be

offensive for handicapped adults. However, I have found that adults as well as children take and use whatever they find of meaning.

(1992: 229)

As the woman from the group explained the members' perspective on the equipment situation to me, I felt completely ashamed of myself for having previously bought into mainstream assumptions about how group members should behave. Of course she was right, and the group should have been given the option to use both sets of equipment. I feel sure that had they not been people with learning difficulties others would not have sought to police their activities in this way. Unfortunately the group's sessions then ended for the summer, and by the time they resumed I had finished the field-work, so I do not know whether the petition succeeded in changing the organizers' minds. Still, this incident taught me a great deal about the strength of my own investments in some of my mainstream identities, and was a salutary lesson about the need for researchers to investigate both sides of an argument, rather than simply accepting the position which best serves our own political purposes.

Individual versus group action

The example given above shows how disabled people at Greenways came together as a group to demand change. I too was given the opportunity to work for change with other disabled people at the site, but I did not always choose to take this option, even though such a decision went against both my political beliefs and my previous professional practice. What happened was this. During my original site access negotiations with James, he had led me to believe that there was an advisory group of disabled people at Greenways that gave feedback to the Centre's management on access issues. He had also suggested that I might wish to become involved with this group as the fieldwork progressed. Although at the outset I was wary of such direct involvement because I felt that it might compromise my position as a 'neutral researcher', as time went on and I developed a range of roles which involved me actively in the life of the Centre, I decided to find out more about this group, and asked James if I could attend one of their meetings. It was then that he told me there was no separate advisory group as such, but that he received occasional feedback on access issues from the staff of the group in which I had already observed the oppressive practice described in the last chapter. In other words, it was not true user feedback at all, but came instead from a source I already had reason to mistrust. On seeing my horrified expression at this revelation, James then said that perhaps I could involve the group members in my own consultancy activities around the site, as a means both of empowering them and of getting more feedback on disabled people's access needs.

He then reinforced his expectation that I would take responsibility for organizing such a group by missing a meeting which we had arranged with them to discuss existing access provision, apparently believing that I would lead it in his absence. In fact, I simply cancelled the meeting, as I was not prepared to work with the staff of that group, or to take sole responsibility for access and customer relations issues which it should have been down to Centre management to deal with.

As a result of my actions, I am all too aware that the group members lost out on an opportunity to make their voices heard in this setting, and that participation in the access auditing process might have helped them develop enough skills and confidence to be able in future to challenge the oppressive practice of their staff. However, I also had to bear in mind why I was conducting this research. At its most basic level, I was there to collect enough data to fulfil my research contract, and any changes to policy and practice which I could help bring about in the process were in that sense merely added bonuses. It is true that I could have involved the group in my work, but before doing so I would have needed to organize additional funding to cover the extra costs of group work, as well as providing them with both assertiveness and audit skills training. This could have added up to a year onto the timescale of the research, and was an additional resource investment I simply could not afford, given the time-limited nature of my own research funding. As a result, I acted selfishly by protecting my research programme at the expense of supporting and giving choices to other disabled people who were undoubtedly more oppressed than me. I am not proud of my actions in this regard, but it is something that I have to live with.

Treating people disrespectfully

Over the course of the fieldwork I came into repeated contact with Daniel, a man with learning difficulties who made it clear from the start of our acquaintance that he wanted to go out with me. However, the need to act as a professional researcher meant I could not afford to give the impression that I was romantically involved with anyone at the site, and so having a relationship with him was never an option. What I am not proud of, however, was the way in which I rejected his sometimes intrusive advances. Unfortunately, I suspect that he had never been given advice about how to chat up women, because he had a tendency both to get very excitable and to invade my personal space while he was talking to me. Once, for example, he came up and loomed right over me as I sat working, effectively trapping me against the table. Although I knew that his intentions were innocent, I still felt helpless and just a bit scared, and in the end when he wouldn't back off I lost my temper and shouted at him to go away. Just then two of the other men from his group came past. Seeing what was going on, they took him gently by the arm and led him away. As they went, I heard them explaining to him that he should not stand so close to people, because they didn't like it. Their patience made me ashamed that I had not acted in a similarly compassionate manner. However, on this occasion I did feel at least partly justified in my actions, in that as a man he was behaving in a way that was oppressive to me as a woman. Nonetheless, I wish that I had not been reduced to ordering him away as if he were some kind of animal, secure in the knowledge that he would obey because of my relative power as someone without learning difficulties. In that respect, it was another example of my potential to abuse someone less powerful than me.

On another occasion when he would not take no for an answer, I again resorted to using every tool at my disposal in order to show him how impossible it was that I would go out with him. I did this by highlighting the differences between us on the basis of my supposed intellectual superiority as someone without learning difficulties. Thus I variously emphasized and invented aspects of my experience to which I knew he himself did not have access, such as being at college, and having a boyfriend who was a teacher, and who also had a big car, and implied that such things mattered to me when deciding who I would go out with. So, even though I like to think of myself as being egalitarian, and as treating other people as I would like to be treated myself, the fact was that in this situation my self-interest was greater still, and I was quite prepared to compromise my social principles in favour of looking out for number one. This incident revealed to me the true and shameful extent of my own social conditioning, and the amount of work I still have to do in working towards inclusive practice.

Some conclusions

In some ways this chapter has been the most difficult for me to write, because it has involved acknowledging something of my own power for evil. The incidents reported here are ones which I would have preferred to have kept hidden, knowing that they do not show me in a good light. Certainly, they lend empirical evidence in support of social model claims (Swain and French, 2000; Vernon, 1999: 389) that each of us has the potential to oppress others who are less powerful than we are. In turn, this suggests that disabled as well as non-disabled people may need to review their current practice, and to look for ways of behaving in a more inclusive manner. Evidence from members of minority groups within the disabled people's movement (Campbell and Oliver, 1996; Stuart, 1993; Vernon, 1996) suggests that this is not always the case at present.

In terms of dealing with non-disabled people, it may be true that disabled people are in less danger of becoming oppressors than of being on the receiving end of oppression. However, in other aspects of our individual identities the power relations involved may not be as straightforward, and as disabled people we need to be aware of our own oppressive potential in those situations. In my own case at Greenways, this did not relate solely to my abuse of people with learning difficulties. For example, it might be argued that, in choosing not to interview four out of the five minority ethnic members of staff, I was behaving in a racist way. Similarly, it was not until I was writing up the results of the fieldwork that it occurred to me to question fully the absence of minority ethnic disabled people from the setting, and to look for reasons for that absence. In addition to un-covering my oppression of people with learning difficulties, then, conducting this research has also made me more aware of the extent of my own racism. In practical terms, too, had I not been forced to review some of my racist beliefs I suspect that I would not have been able to develop such a good working relationship with James, or to in turn be in a position to influence some of the subsequent access initiatives at the site. Hence I believe that challenging our own prejudices is important not just in abstract social justice terms, but also in practical ways, in opening up the possibility of forming alliances for change with previously unconsidered partners. Some of the ways in which I attempted to do this at Greenways are discussed in the next chapter.

Chapter 13

Being an activist

Activism and research: a dilemma for disabled researchers

Juggling the roles of ethnographer and action researcher was a central activity throughout my time at Greenways but mostly, whichever role I was occupying, I managed to retain a good-enough professional distance between myself and the participants. So, for example, I pointed out to the management some areas where I felt that staff or customers were being treated unfairly, but I was careful to couch my comments in relatively neutral terms and to avoid my intervention being seen as a crusade. However, there were some instances during the research – especially in my identity as a disabled person – where neutrality was not an option, and where I had to become actively involved in a partisan way that might be considered to have gone beyond the boundaries usually associated with conducting academic research. This chapter discusses those instances, together with one occasion where I was unhappy with what I was seeing, but did not act. I have included this example because one of the most valuable lessons which undertaking this research has taught me is that activism is partly about choosing which battles to fight, and recognizing that some may be just too difficult to take on at that particular time and place.

More widely, the purpose of this chapter is to address the issue of how far disabled researchers should be expected to go in the course of their work. Sometimes in the field of disability studies there seems to be an expectation that disabled researchers will inevitably also be activists, and that they will be prepared to endure unpleasant reminders of their own oppression in the course of conducting their fieldwork because in research terms the project is seen as being more important than they are. Too often I have heard non-disabled researchers, in response to disabled researchers' harrowing accounts of dealing with fieldwork oppression, say things like 'what a fascinating piece of research'. Well, yes, it might be, but actually such a superficial response to real researcher pain is not adequate. In fact, it is frankly insulting, when for many disabled people participation in disability research can never be a neutral act, but one in which they may be implicated heart and soul, and which may cause them great suffering as a result. Similarly, some non-disabled researchers have told me of their own distress at having been unable to give as much support to their own research participants as they would have liked. Perhaps, then, disabled people's experience is indicative of a more general concern within the research community at being torn between the academic and fund-holder demands associated with the research process, and a personal desire for accountability towards the groups and individuals with whom the research is conducted (Goodley and Moore, 2000).

In my own case, having a research support group to help me deal with some of the things I witnessed at Greenways was crucially important. Even so, I had some bad experiences where nobody else could follow me and help me through, and where it had to be down to me to sort it out. At those times, being an activist was something of a double bind. The social model gave me a political focus and showed me what I had to do to resolve those situations, but at the same time it made me all too aware of instances of oppression I might otherwise have been able to avoid confronting. What helped me to retain some sense of perspective at such times was the memory of what a colleague once said to me about the early feminists. He told me that they did a marvellous job of uncovering and deconstructing women's oppression, but that in the process they gave so much of themselves that many of them either died young or dropped out. He said, and I agree with him, that our task as second- and third-generation activists is to bring about change without destroying ourselves in the process, otherwise any progress made is likely to be a Pyrrhic victory. What follows is an account of my attempts to put this principle into practice in my research at Greenways.

Advantages and disadvantages of being an activist at Greenways

From the very start of this research, there was an expectation among Greenways staff that my study would identify areas where changes were needed to make the Centre more accessible. In previous chapters I have discussed some of the ways in which I fulfilled this expectation through policy document analysis, access auditing, the preparation of a thirty-point action plan of suggested access improvements, and my final consultancy report recommending changes to policy and practice within the organization. Here I want to focus less on those measurable outcomes than on how it felt for me to be cast in – and to almost always unquestioningly accept – such a figurehead activist role. In many ways I was happy to fall into a slot with which I was familiar, and in which I knew that I could deliver the goods. Yet there were also disadvantages to it, especially where I saw things happening which I could not approve of, and/or which reminded me all too powerfully of past instances of my own oppression. Sometimes, too, the activist role seemed to conflict directly with those of being a researcher and a member of staff, and there were times where I was sure that my advice was being ignored in favour of maintaining the status quo. In those cases I felt particularly uncomfortable, in case my continued presence at the site was seen as sanctioning bad practice.

My identity as a disabled person was fundamentally implicated here. Although it facilitated my activist role in much the same way as James could when necessary use his identity as a 'black expert', such a role also places extra demands on the individual, as he points out here:

> . . . being black then, it gives me a lever at times, to say 'that's wrong' or 'this is what you need to do'. Very difficult sometimes, especially if you've got someone who's supposed to be in a minority group, but has got the confidence, the ability and education and the facts, to be able to argue with you. It can be very, very powerful. So that aspect of it. And the other thing that being black also has helped me to be able to challenge things. Because there's an expectation that I will, because I always have done, and to progress you have to – you can't just sit down and say 'I'm not interested' or 'I don't like it'. You have to have an opinion, and that opinion is sought after at times, if not (always) used as it should be.

By the same token, at Greenways I felt that I had a responsibility towards other disabled people to report access barriers to the management, and to attempt to influence change. However, as I have said above, there were times when my advice went unheeded. For example, there was an ongoing failure to police illegal parking in the 'disabled only' zone, and to rectify even relatively minor access barriers, such as re-hanging toilet doors so that they opened outwards instead of inwards to improve access for wheelchair users. Particularly where such barriers had been reported to me by other disabled people, I felt that I was letting my brothers and sisters down by failing to bring about change. Instead I allowed myself to be bought off with assurances that improvements would be made once the Centre was refurbished. However, two years on this refurbishment has still not taken place, and so many access barriers remain. Conscious of the need to avoid being seen as a token 'disability expert', I had also put the management in touch with the local disabled people's organization, in the hope that ongoing alliances and working partnerships might be developed in that way. However, subsequent feedback from this group suggests that nothing concrete has been achieved to date. There were, then, a number of occasions when I felt my presence was used to give the illusion rather than the reality that the organization was committed to change. I do not wish to paint too much of a conspiracy theory picture here, because I know that some of the staff I worked with were extremely frustrated that a lack of corporate funding and/or low prioritization of access improvement work meant that they could not implement all of my recommendations immediately as they would have liked. However, as James has suggested, it will probably not be until leisure organizations attach the same level of importance to community development initiatives as they do to income generation that change will come.

More positively, I was told that my feedback to Greenways had been at least partly responsible for an organizational decision to create a new corporate-level community development post to develop better links with community groups and encourage more people to use the leisure facilities on offer across the town. As a result, issues such as the underrepresentation of disabled and minority ethnic people in leisure activities now receive more attention than before. Such structural changes are important steps in the right direction, and in this case have led to the implementation of some of my research recommendations, including the introduction of a new pricing policy which gives disabled people discounted entry to all leisure centres in the town, plus free entry to an essential support worker. This development suggests that individuals working from social model principles can act as catalysts to bring about wider structural change.

Choosing not to act

In Chapter 11 I discussed my experience of disabling prejudice in my interactions with a local council worker when we met at a junior basketball tournament held at the Centre. Here, I want to expand on that discussion by looking at the tournament and my objections to it in more detail, together with the reasons why I chose not to take a stand against it at the time. Originally it was James who told me that a wheelchair basketball event was going to take place, and he suggested that it might be useful for my research if I were to go along and observe what went on. However, as previously discussed he failed to tell me in advance that the event was not a true wheelchair basketball tournament, but was instead primarily a simulation exercise designed to give non-disabled children the chance to try out the sport, with the hoped-for by-product that this experience would in future make them more tolerant of disabled people. The event had received grant aid from a prestigious national organization, which increased its credibility as a 'worthy cause', and which in turn probably accounted for the presence of the local mayor and other civic dignitaries on the day.

There were a number of specific things about the event to which I objected. First, that it was being held at all, when I could see little practical benefit accruing from it in terms of changing people's attitudes towards disabled people in the real world, especially since only one of the organizers and one of the participants were disabled people. Second, I noted that participation in an activity with a disability theme seemed to give the non-disabled organizers the right to leave their cars in the reserved disabled people's car park, thus reducing real disabled people's access to such spaces. Third, as reported previously, being involved in a charitable event seemed to make some people feel that they could act in a patronizing and oppressive way towards me. Points two and three taken together thus suggest that many of the organizers, at least, were learning nothing from their involvement in this project about how to treat disabled people with respect. Fourth, and perhaps most gallingly, I noted that the participants had been given high performance sports chairs to use during the event. Yet at the same time anecdotal evidence suggested that there were real disabled people living in that town who were being refused access to the high-quality wheelchairs they needed for daily living, apparently on cost grounds. I simply could not see what was right about giving non-disabled people access to high-quality impairment-related equipment when it was being denied to the people who really needed it.

For me the episode reinforced the dangers of promoting awareness-raising simulation activities which, besides being unrealistic, often fail to incorporate discussion of the reality of the wider political environment. In mitigation, it must be said that the one disabled person who was involved in organizing the event told me that he felt the children taking part did learn from the experience, and that they acted more inclusively towards disabled people as a result. However, the oppressive behaviour I experienced from some of his colleagues, together with the complete lack of wider political awareness shown in staging such an event, left me unconvinced of the effectiveness of such activities as a means of countering discrimination. For me, the event served primarily as an example of the gap between old-style disability awareness training as still used in some areas of sport and recreation, and the newer, less exploitative disability equality training, which has abandoned the use of simulation exercises in favour of employing real disabled people to tell it like it is. The basketball experience was thus a salutary reminder of what we are up against in seeking to bring about change. Frankly, I was left with the feeling that the main people to benefit from this particular event were the non-disabled organizers, who clearly felt pleased with themselves for being seen to be 'doing good' through their involvement in a recognizably charitable activity.

Despite my objections, however, I did not actively challenge the event organizers about their objectives at the time. In taking this decision, it was not that I didn't have enough well-developed arguments to use against them, but was instead simply a question of numbers. There were between fifty and seventy people at the event who seemed quite happy with what was going on, and only one of me. As a result I felt completely overwhelmed, particularly after I was on the receiving end of oppression from some of the organizers. This robbed me of my ability to feel strong and proud, and left me depressed to think of just how much prejudice we have to counter in this world. At the time, then, it could be said that I did not take action by default, because the situation neutralized my identity and made me powerless. Later, I discussed the incident with my support group, and we looked at the possibility of several of us attending the same activity together another time, so that I would be properly supported and could then more effectively challenge the way in which the event was organized. In the end, however, I decided against doing this, since for the purposes of my research I had already collected enough useful data the first time around. The sole purpose of a return visit would have been to try to bring about change, an endeavour which I suspected the entrenched positions of some of the organizers would have made very difficult to achieve. Further, this activity had little direct impact on service provision for real disabled people at the Centre. Apart from restating to James my objections to the use of simulation exercises, I therefore chose not to take any further action in this case. It felt like too big a battle to take on at that time.

Forming alliances for change

In the past, I have usually dealt with instances of oppressive practice in one of two ways. Either, as shown above, I have felt powerless to respond, or else I have 'gone it alone' in a self-styled personal crusade against injustice. Sometimes the latter approach works, but it has usually left me exhausted as a result. However, at Greenways my position as a relatively powerless unpaid researcher (in contrast to the paid, officially sanctioned, members of staff) meant that I could not personally enforce any changes within the setting, but instead could only put forward a case to persuade others to act. In terms of much of my work there I could deal with this, since it was not all that different from being a consultant, in that you might offer people advice but you could not force them to take it. However, some of the incidents which I observed at Greenways required a more involved and personal response, especially when it came to confronting the abusive staff behaviour I witnessed in one segregated group, and which I have previously discussed in Chapter 11.

Initially in this particular case I was at a loss to know how to react, even though my observational studies of this group, together with my support worker's confirmation that the staff's behaviour was not acceptable, made me realise that I could not pretend to be a neutral observer and stand by and do nothing. However, to begin with I was crushed by a whole range of emotions which included despair that such abuse was still going on at the start of the twenty-first century, pain and inconsolable grief at what I was witnessing, fury to think that the staff were getting away with such behaviour, and fear of what might happen to the group members if I took action and reported the staff. My relative lack of power within the situation also made me conscious that there might actually be little that I could do to bring about change. As a result my mind was in turmoil, and my indecision was particularly enhanced by the knowledge that any action I did decide to take might have serious repercussions for the group members.

In the end, my research supervisor's intervention proved crucial to moving things forward. When I asked him what to do, he simply told me that some issues are too big to deal with on your own, and that all I could do in this situation was to tell James what was going on, and let him take it from there. To be honest, I was not too sure about doing this, because I had all sorts of emotional barriers in place against revealing too much of the pain around disabling practice to a non-disabled person who at that point I did not know very well. Despite what I said in Chapter 10 about the need for greater openness between disabled and non-disabled people, this case was so personal and potentially so dangerous that it did indeed feel too much like making private matters into public issues. I also could not be sure that James would take my complaint seriously. After all, he might be black, but he was also non-disabled, and had more power than me within that setting. Perhaps he would refuse to listen to what I had to say, and would choose instead to side with other authority figures in the shape of the very staff I wanted to complain about. Additionally, the idea of forming an alliance to tackle such a sensitive disability issue with a non-disabled person was frightening to me, given my previous preference for working alone or with other disabled people on such matters. Yet when it came down to it, I realised that I had no choice but to try to trust James if I wanted to see things change.

In the event, as reported in Chapter 11, I found that as soon as I made my opening, deliberately vague, comment about not being sure that the group were making the best possible use of the facilities, he responded by detailing his own concerns about what was going on there. As I concluded previously, it seemed that he had needed my 'expert' confirmation that what was going on was wrong, before he could take action. However, once he was clear about that, and we had discussed what the options were, he took action to try to put things right. It then became a hidden partnership between us. Aware of the emotional and power-relational conflicts which made it impossible for me to take a public role in challenging the staff concerned, he acted as front man, but at each stage we would get together afterwards to discuss their responses, and to decide what he should do next.

Thus he started off by telling Dominic, the group leader, that he was not happy about the way the group was being run, and in particular about the amount of time that people spent sitting passively in a separate room rather than taking part in Centre activities. Dominic's response was to claim that he didn't have enough staff to support group members in other activities (although actually staffing was almost one to one), following this up by saying that they did not have enough money to pay for extra sports sessions anyway. James responded by offering free entry to those extra activities, and also suggested another meeting with the group to discuss any access concerns they might have. We subsequently discovered that Dominic reported this suggestion back to the group as a complaint by James against them as members, and as a threat to withdraw use of all facilities from them – so needless to say, no such meeting took place.

At this point we realized that we were up against someone who appeared prepared to deflect blame from himself and onto others. Unaware of my concerns about the way he was running the group, he even tried to involve me on his side, by asking me to complain to James about access provision at the site. I realized then that we had not taken sufficient account of the strength of Dominic's psychological investments in keeping things as they were, nor of the power relations that enabled him to do so. In retrospect, this made me wish that I had read Brown's analysis of the response of vulnerable staff to unwelcome change before we tackled him. Brown suggests that:

> In this case, staff are likely to become more rigid when their power is challenged, to grip on to the authoritarian responses which they learned from observation and to wipe out the potential to identify with the people who are on the receiving end of their oppressive behaviour.
>
> (1992: 194)

For me, this sums up Dominic's response to our intervention perfectly. As soon as his behaviour was challenged, he resorted to putting the blame elsewhere – onto James, the group, and a supposed lack of staff and funding. At no stage did he accept personal responsibility for the failure of adequate service provision. His seeming attempts at manipulation were fairly transparent, but his actions were still potentially damaging, because he had the power to deny services to the group. Had I been aware in advance that his behaviour was likely to follow such a pattern, I might have decided either to act more openly and forcefully myself, or to have reported him to social services. However, the further progression of events suggested that this might have had limited results. As the months progressed there were some improvements, in that the group did start to participate in more Centre activities. However, the relationship between the Centre and Dominic continued to deteriorate, until eventually a meeting was held with the group and Dominic's manager, at which – predictably – he tried to blame James for everything. Unsurprisingly, James told me that none of the other staff or the group members supported these claims. However, whilst Dominic's manager seemed concerned at what he heard, no action was taken against him, and at the time when I finished the research he was still in charge of the group, although I understand that he has since left to work in another field.

In some respects, the patchy nature of the changes made in that group as a result of the alliance between James and me could be seen as a failure. Certainly we did not achieve everything that we set out to do at the time, although it was not a total disaster because some changes did take place both then and later. At another level too, our partnership was a valuable learning experience for me. Through it I learned that I did not always have to tackle oppression by myself, and that it was possible to trust at least some non-disabled people to do the right thing in challenging disabling practices.

In the fieldwork as a whole, the mix of skills and experience which James and I brought to our working partnership was also crucial. Acting alone I would not have had the same power to bring about changes in the setting, while he needed my specific experience of dealing with disablist oppression to guide his action and thus make it more effective. Our ability to work together was based on our having sufficient commonality in elements of our multiple identities to recognize that an alliance between us was possible. It is important to note, though, that in other situations we might not have chosen such a partnership. As Bagihole explains in terms of the experience of black women fighting oppression:

> (she) might need to fight racism at one point and sexism at another time, and at other times the sexism she is fighting is tainted and influenced by racism. Her allies may change in these different fights and so might her strategy. The dynamic mix of sexism, racism and disablism demands different reactions at different times and in different contexts.
>
> (1997: 41)

In terms of my research at Greenways, however, James was the best situational ally I could hope for. Linked in terms of our class, professional backgrounds and personalities, we also had experiences of oppression that allowed us to make connections with each other and to fight disablism in that setting. By the end things had improved compared to how they were when the fieldwork began, and there was the promise of further change once the improvements to policy and practice which I had recommended were put in place. All in all, then, I was able to leave the field feeling that I had done the best that I could in the circumstances.

Some conclusions

In this chapter I have tried to show something of the intensity of the emotional and moral conflicts which I, as a disabled person and as a researcher, had to deal with at Greenways, and which I could sometimes only confront by taking direct action to influence change. It should be clear from my comments that these were issues which at times threatened to overwhelm me, and which I would have been unable to cope with had it not been for the back-up of my research supervisor, my support group and James. I hope that in this respect my experiences may serve as further justification of the need for institutional support for (in this case) disabled researchers, so that unlike the early feminists they come through such experiences suffering no long-term ill effects, and able to apply their skills to future research projects.

As I have also explained, my experience of influencing change at Greenways was inextricably linked to the need to recognize the various ways in which power relations operated there, and the understanding that I would therefore need to form situational alliances with other people who were more powerful than me in order to challenge existing disabling practice. In one sense, this strategy could refer to all my relationships with non-disabled people there, and certainly I remain mindful of the remark reported in Chapter 9 about the need for disabled people to be more open about sharing examples of our oppression with them if we want non-disabled people to support us in our struggles. Often, too, such alliances did not just benefit me. For example, James did not need me to fight his battles against racism for him, but there were occasions when we discussed situations he was having to deal with, and it is hoped that my support was useful to him at those times.

More generally, I feel that my activist experience at Greenways was a practical example of what Finkelstein meant when he called on disabled people to become involved in wider struggles for change alongside non-disabled people (1996: 11). This is a principle which I practised here primarily through my advocacy of staff concerns to the management about the impact on them of the company's reorganization. However, the development of my alliance with James to bring about change also highlighted some key issues that may be implicated for members of minority groups in seeking to work with others in this way. In particular, in this instance there was the need to first develop trust between the parties and to know that we each implicitly believed what the other was saying, together with the pragmatic recognition of the potential impact of existing power relations on an individual or group's ability to take action. If James had not understood how these factors impacted on me in this setting, then we would not have been able to work together so effectively.

This chapter concludes my analysis of the data collected at Greenways. In the final chapter, I summarize my main findings and attempt to draw some wider conclusions from the research.

Chapter 14

Conclusions

Researching the interface between disabled and non-disabled people

In this book I have explored some aspects of non-disabled people's constructions of disability, as revealed through a study of their interactions with disabled people at Greenways Leisure Centre. In researching the interface in this way, I discovered that a combination of structural and attitudinal factors appeared to affect the potential for inclusion in this setting. Generally speaking, those disabled people who visited the Centre independently appeared to receive the same level of service as other customers, and were seen as ordinary participants by staff and other users. Being treated as ordinary in this way seemed to depend on disabled people's willingness to take part in the activities on offer, and in going swimming or working out alongside non-disabled people the commonality of the activity appeared to take priority over any bodily differences.

However, the research has also shown that many disabled people who visited Greenways as part of large segregated groups did not experience inclusion in this way, but instead remained the objects of negative stereotyping which portrayed them as 'other'. Data indicate that non-disabled people saw them as being frightening, different and requiring separate leisure provision which served the additional purpose of keeping them under surveillance. I have suggested that non-disabled people's failure to move beyond seeing group members in these negatively stereotypical ways resulted principally from the structural barrier of offering primarily large-scale segregated leisure provision, especially to people with learning difficulties, and staffing such groups with external contractors who brought assumptions of disabled people's deficit on the grounds of impairment into this more inclusive setting. At Greenways, possible solutions to this problem include involving the Centre's own staff in the running of segregated groups, and encouraging more disabled people to visit individually or in much smaller groups in the future. While wholesale segregated leisure provision for people with learning difficulties remains the norm, it is hard to see how they will be able to discover any commonality between their experiences and those of non-disabled people, and vice versa.

Further, the research findings also suggest that even for those disabled people who did join mainstream activity sessions, full inclusion was not always guaranteed. For example, my interviews with the non-disabled staff revealed that they were operating on assumptions of a hierarchy of impairment, with wheelchair users being seen as 'real disabled people', and all ambulant disabled people being classed as 'normal' or 'almost normal'. In this sports setting, then, an ability to walk was seen by the staff as the main differential between disabled and non-disabled people. In turn this also suggested a general lack of awareness of the access needs of the much larger customer group comprising ambulant disabled people. There also appeared to be a related perception that high-level functional ability was the key prerequisite of disabled people being able to join in with mainstream activities, even though this ran contrary to some empirical evidence, including that of my own participation. This in turn was 'explained' by the staff in terms of my supposed higher level of confidence, and a stated perception that my impairment was 'less severe' than those of other disabled people at the site – even though this was not always the case. One possible explanation for this is that, as one of my friends has suggested, some of the staff needed to name me as 'special', 'different' or 'less severe than' other disabled people so that they could justify to themselves why it was that they could be with me and have a good time, 'even though' I'm a disabled person. She thought that if they did not try to justify singling me out in this way, it would mean they would have to have to allow for the possibility that they could – if they were to change their exclusionary mindset – have equally good relationships with other disabled people. This explanation makes a lot of sense to me. It reveals the pernicious extent of negative social conditioning against disabled people as a group, and shows just how far even those people who demonstrate otherwise good practice towards particular individuals have to go before they can truly be deemed to be acting inclusively.

During the research I also noted the routine use of out-of-date terminology to describe disabled people and disabled people's experience, with phrases such as 'confined to a wheelchair' and 'mentally handicapped' being routinely used by leisure staff at interview. Overall, therefore, in pondering on whether we may need to develop a common language with non-disabled 'others' before being able to discuss disability issues, the data certainly suggest that we don't always have one at present. Nobody at Greenways used the term 'impairment' or referred to the social model, which suggests that the disabled people's movement has not yet managed to publicize its preferred terminology or ideas to a wider audience beyond that directly involved in disability issues. This also suggests that there is scope for the marketing of disability equality training courses in more sport and leisure settings, to explain how social model ideas can be used to help develop more inclusive policies and practices. However, conducting the research has also shown me that challenging exclusion is not just a question of language. It is also about a need to get people to question their automatic assumptions about disabled people needing to be looked after or kept in one place, which is about differential and negative treatment. When Centre staff saw outside 'professional carers' treating disabled people differently, it was little wonder that they assumed such behaviour to be necessary and right, especially since they were unaware of the apparent psychoanalytic imperatives at work in some disability professionals who spend all their working lives defending against the 'horror' of impairment, leading them to act abusively towards disabled people as a result. In such ways is exclusionary behaviour tolerated and sustained. Even James needed to hear from me that members of one of the groups were being abused before he would take action, although he has since admitted that he would only need to have seen similar behaviour once towards non-disabled children to have taken action. All this hints at a gulf in understanding, with disabled people (especially those who visited Greenways in groups) being automatically seen as incompetent 'others', or as having different, and lesser, values and aspirations than do people in the mainstream. So in fact, the persistence of disablist practice at Greenways resulted from a combination of factors. It was about language and power and negative role models (among 'professional carers') and assumptions of incompetence in 'othered' groups. No one of these factors was primary at all times.

Of course, it should go without saying that because this research was on a small scale and was based only in one setting, it would be wrong to suggest that its findings can be universally applied elsewhere. However, I do believe that in interrogating the experience of inclusion and exclusion for disabled people at Greenways this study has served a useful purpose, not least in revealing the impossibility of trying to understand events in this one setting in isolation from the wider social, cultural, economic and political environment of which it is a part. Thus, despite its acknowledged limitations of scale, it is hoped that some of the research findings will be of use to others who are working towards inclusive practice, either as practitioners, or as theoreticians, or both.

Practitioner-related research conclusions

In documenting the range of leisure provision offered to disabled people at Greenways, the research has identified a number of steps that both the site's leisure managers and the contracted disability service providers could take to make their services more inclusive.

For the leisure managers, the following structural changes were recommended. These should be read within the wider context of the need to comply with Part III of the 1995 Disability Discrimination Act, which covers access to goods and services. At Greenways, then, this might be achieved in some of the following ways. The organization could produce information about the Centre's leisure activities in alternative formats (e.g. in large print, on tape, and taped in other community languages) to reach a wider market audience; ensure that all public areas of the sites are well-lit, and that directional signage using good colour contrast is placed where people with visual impairments can get close up to read it and so be able to find their way around independently; install hearing induction loops at reception points and in teaching areas, and reduce the use of background music in sessions attended by people with hearing impairments, so that they are more likely to pick up on what the session leader is saying; arrange for session leaders to be given disability equality training to increase their awareness of disabled people's needs; and offer discounted entry prices for disabled people and any essential support worker. In addition, from 2004 any such programme access changes will also need to be supplemented by 'reasonable adjustments' to physical access at the site. This might include addressing other barriers highlighted by this research, such as the need to properly police accessible parking bays reserved for disabled people; re-hanging toilet doors so they open outwards and thus make the toilets more wheelchair-accessible; replacing the heavy front doors with automatic ones; and replacing the 'gravel trap' carpets in some areas of the Centre with ones with a shallower tread. It should be noted that a number of these suggested physical and programme improvements would involve little additional cost to the organization, and are expected to be beneficial in terms of attracting a wider range of customers to the site, thus helping to generate more income. Further, none of these changes would limit or damage the service provided to existing Centre users. Indeed, those concerned with providing information in alternative formats such as on tape and in community languages might be expected to increase the Centre's appeal to an even wider customer market, including people from minority ethnic groups, and the 20 per cent of the population who have limited literacy skills (Department for Education and Skills, 1999) and who might also therefore welcome receiving information in a verbal format that they can more easily understand. This shows that services provided initially with disabled people's needs in mind can help to create the potential for inclusion for other groups as well.

In addition to these general findings, other recommendations arising out of the research relate specifically to the segregated activity sessions offered to disabled people at Greenways. These may be of interest to both leisure managers and to disability service providers in other leisure settings. First, the research suggests that all staff who organize and run segregated leisure activities for disabled people should be skilled in leisure service provision, and should be bound by the leisure centre's own equal opportunities policies. Ideally, these segregated sessions should be run by the leisure centre's own staff, both to raise the standard of teaching and to increase the possibilities for inclusion. Second, leisure sessions organized for disabled people should be staffed with enough support workers so that participants have the opportunity to get changed into sports clothes, and to receive appropriate levels of individual support during the activity. Third, segregated activity sessions should be limited to a maximum of ten participants, and those smaller sessions might then be offered across the week. This would enable more effective teaching, and by reducing non-disabled people's fear of large groups of disabled people would further increase the possibilities for inclusion. Fourth, segregated activities can and should be a starting point from which people go on to participate in mainstream sessions, with appropriate support where necessary. Thus the introduction of discounted pricing policies like that at Greenways may be expected to further facilitate disabled people's opportunities to take part in mainstream leisure centre activities. Finally, all staff working with disabled people should be offered both disability equality training and, where appropriate, activity-specific training to enable them to deliver their sessions to a wider range of customers.

As I have indicated, some of the recommendations made in the previous paragraph are relevant to the work of disability service providers as well as to leisure managers. In addition, in supporting normalization/SRV critiques of unacceptable service provision (Brown and Smith, 1992; Race, 1999; Wolfensberger, 1992) the research has identified some ways in which existing disability service provision at Greenways could be modified in order to increase the potential for inclusion. In particular, it has shown how the current mass group provision of leisure activities for disabled people, combined with poor staffing levels and inappropriate behaviour by some group leaders, devalued customers with learning difficulties in a way that mainstream services at the site did not. This was a particularly worrying research finding, suggesting that staff who work with disabled people *must* learn to see disabled people as ordinary members of society who deserve access to the same level and quality of service as they would expect for themselves. At present, however, it seemed that many were unable to do this, thereby perpetuating an impression that disabled customers had no right to expect anything better than what they were being offered. Further, disabled people who attended these groups often appeared to have no real opportunity to complain about the services they received; and when James and I did try to take action to improve provision in one group this was strongly resisted by the group leader. Some of these 'spoiling tactics' may in turn have derived from inadequate training and support provision for these community-based disability staff, leading them instead to fall back on individualized defensive coping strategies that further reinforced disabled people's powerlessness. Thus the research has highlighted the need previously identified by Smith and Brown (1992) for community-based service staff to receive proper ongoing support and training to deal with the stress associated with their jobs. In the meantime, it appeared that what we might call 'institutional disablism' among some of these disability service providers was a major factor in perpetuating the exclusion of (in particular) people with learning difficulties in this setting. It is to be hoped that such issues of power and control will begin to be addressed through the further development of normalization/SRV theory around the effect of power relations on service provision, which in turn may be expected to lead to improved training for disability staff, perhaps through initiatives like the new Learning Difficulty Awards Framework (Department of Health, 2001). Most important of all, such changes may – indeed must – result in a better standard of service for disabled people.

Research conclusions relating to normalization/SRV theory

In the previous section I suggested that my research findings indicate that normalization/SRV theory needs to engage more systematically than it has previously done with issues of power and control, in order to improve service provision for disabled people. Certainly at Greenways it was at once interesting and terrifying to note that the power of the disability professionals went unchallenged by most of the leisure staff, simply because they assumed that those professionals were always acting in the best interests of the group members. This suggests that it may be dangerous for normalization/SRV theorists to argue that community-based services may in themselves provide a check on abusive behaviour by disability staff, because of the increased potential for intervention of other members of the community to prevent abuse (Race, 1999). Instead, in this setting I have demonstrated that the 'disability professional' identity appeared in the eyes of the leisure services staff to be all-powerful, and so no action to prevent further abuse was taken until I intervened. It is interesting to speculate whether such behaviour would be more likely to be challenged by members of the wider leisure centre community if it were to happen now, in the post Harold Shipman era where medical and care professionals are no longer accorded the same unquestioned levels of deference and respect as they were at the time of this research. Certainly, I hope this would be the case. However, a more effective way of tackling abuse by disability staff would be to sack those responsible, and to develop a more systematic theory-level approach to tackling oppressive power relations that can then be used to support the development of more inclusive policies and practices.

The research also highlighted what is for me another limitation in the potential of normalization/SRV theory to support disabled people's wider social inclusion. The 'conservatism corollary' approach recommended by Wolfensberger (1992) suggests that disabled people should do all they can to minimize their visible difference from normative standards of appearance and behaviour, in order to 'pass' (Goffman, 1990) as normal. However, even if disabled people were prepared to compromise the impairment-related parts of their identity in this way, the data presented here suggest that such an approach can never be completely successful. As I discovered myself while at Greenways, the fact that I occupied the socially valued roles of researcher, consultant, member of staff, and so on did not protect me from oppression in all situations. Similarly, although James was both a high-level leisure manager and a sporting celebrity, he too faced daily racist oppression. Thus full assimilation on the basis of our approximation to normative standards of appearance and behaviour was simply not possible, because at the end of the day he was a black man and I was a disabled woman, and no amount of dissembling would change the fact that we face ongoing discrimination on the basis of those aspects of our identities. In these circumstances, it was our responses to that ongoing process that was the key both to the maintenance of our self-esteem and to our social survival. For both of us, the assimilation route was not acceptable. Instead, embracing those apparently socially devalued aspects of our identities was the only logical approach, because it enabled us to be proud of who we are, as we are, rather than attempting to engage in a constant struggle for self-regulation in the hope that we might just get away with fitting in as a result. This supports the point that others have previously made about the value of membership of social movements as a means of challenging oppression (Aspis, 2002; Szivos, 1992; Walmsley, 1997). Ultimately, therefore, I believe that disabled people's best hope of achieving real social inclusion lies not in struggling to comply with existing unrealistic normative standards, but rather in embracing all aspects of our identities, including those that the mainstream currently see as being socially devalued, and demanding acceptance on the basis of the equal valuing of difference. I will return to this point later.

Research conclusions relating to social model explanations for disability

As with the application of normalization/SRV theory, the research indicated some conflicting findings around how far the social model can explain what goes on in the disabled/non-disabled interface. Sometimes the data supported existing social model explanations for disabled people's inclusion and exclusion, but elsewhere they uncovered areas of apparent contradiction between theory and practice, as well as highlighting some areas where people's experiences have to date been undertheorized. To start with the positives, the data supported social model theory in the following respects.

First, it supports the emphasis in materialist social model accounts on the need for structural change as a prerequisite for achieving greater social inclusion for disabled people. Such accounts provided real practical guidance for the consultancy element of this fieldwork, and led to suggestions for structural changes at Greenways which included improving physical access, introducing subsidized charges to mainstream activities for disabled people, producing Centre information in accessible formats, and making organizational anti-discrimination policies more consistent. Second, the data also gave practical examples of the ways in which structural change can lead to attitude change, as shown by the contrast between the relatively inclusive behaviour of Centre staff towards disabled people, and the exclusionary approach taken by some of the external contract staff who were not bound by the same anti-discrimination policies. At a basic economic level, staff who relied on the Centre for their main income could not afford to display routinely disabling attitudes, in case they lost their jobs as a result. Third, it supports Oliver's contention (1990: 90–1) that disability professionals do rely on disabled people for their jobs and that, as Chapters 11 and 13 showed, this dependency is often obscured by practices designed to further disempower disabled people. As a result of such actions, disabled people continue to be denied full citizenship (Barton, 1993: 235–6), here demonstrated in ways such as not being able to get changed into appropriate clothing before participating in sporting activities, and not having real choices either to challenge or change the services they are being offered (Aspis, 1997, 2002).

Fourth, the data support calls for the inclusion of an explanation of impairment into the social model to avoid ignoring the reality of the impaired body, and to instead follow mainstream sociological theory in viewing the body as a potential site of resistance to externally imposed ideas and practices (Giddens, 1991; Hughes and Paterson, 1997: 330). Equally I hope that the data presented here have shown something of the pride which I and others in the setting had in our identity as disabled people, and the sense in which our active participation in sport and leisure was an act of affirmation of our impaired bodies (Hughes and Paterson, 1997: 332; Swain and French, 2000). However, I believe that it would be preferable for discussion of impairment to be included in mainstream sociological theory, rather than for a separate theory of impairment to be developed that might only be accessed by disability studies theorists. I am aware that such a suggestion may be difficult to implement, given that much mainstream theory currently draws on the individual/medical model of disability for its analysis. However, I believe that engaging in debate with mainstream theorists, as some disability studies scholars are already doing (for example, Barnes, Mercer and Shakespeare, 1999; Thomas, 1999) is a vital strategic step towards finding common ground on which to discuss these issues and to move towards the development of more inclusive theories in the future. Fifth, the data supported feminist arguments that discussing aspects of disabled people's personal experience may be crucial in exposing existing oppressive practices (Morris, 1991; Thomas, 1999). For example, my experience as a researcher in this setting was conditioned by my personal experience of impairment, and some common research practices were disabling to me because I needed more time, or more support to achieve them, than were automatically available to me. Although initially I was tempted not to discuss these personal issues in this book, they did have a real impact on my ability to conduct the research. I then realized that unless such issues are brought out in the open, and their relationship to wider structural barriers is discussed, their disabling potential will remain (Thomas, 1999: 74).

Sixth, data showed the existence in the setting of multiple and sometimes simultaneous oppressions (Stuart, 1993), especially in relation to women and members of minority ethnic groups, while specific examples presented in Chapter 12 supported the view (Swain and French, 2000: 570; Vernon, 1999) that those conventionally seen as oppressed may themselves oppress other people who have even less power than they do. Taken together, these data support the need identified by Banton and Hirsch (2000), Humphrey (2000), Priestley (1995: 165) and Vernon (1996, 1999) for the disabled people's movement in Britain both to become more inclusive by recognizing the gender, racial and cultural diversity of its membership, and to acknowledge the need of some subgroups of disabled people (for example, members of the gay and lesbian and minority ethnic communities) to organize separately from the mainstream movement on occasion. Finally, the evidence of my successful working partnership with James supported Vernon's (1999: 389) case in favour of the opportunities which the experience of shifting and simultaneous oppressions may provide for the development of alliances with members of other groups, for example by black disabled people with black non-disabled people, or as in our case between a black non-disabled man and a white disabled woman.

In other ways, however, the data critiqued existing social model accounts. First, the interconnectedness of structural and attitudinal barriers uncovered at Greenways suggests a need to question whether structural barriers explanations for disabled people's exclusion are wholly adequate to explain how disability was being constructed there. My contention is rather that neither purely economic nor purely attitudinal explanations for that exclusion are adequate. At the conclusion to this research even more than at the beginning, I am convinced that social model writers must engage more systematically with the problem of disabling attitude barriers in the future. Precisely because such attitudes may be nebulous and intangible, they are in many respects more insidious and pervasive than structural barriers. This suggests that the current undertheorizing of the effects of oppressive attitudes on disabled people is dangerous, because it allows this aspect of disabled people's oppression to remain unduly individualized, and/or analysed only by traditional quantitative attitudes research methodologies that tend to view the individual in isolation from the wider society of which they are a part (Eagly and Chaiken, 1993; Fishbein and Azjen, 1975; Warren and Jahoda, 1976). In my view, therefore, social model writers should not view an increased emphasis on changing attitudes as a dangerous distraction from the main thrust of the most influential arguments of the social model, but should instead follow Thomas (1999) and post-structuralists in incorporating social constructionist and social creationist responses to this very real aspect of disabled people's oppression. Second, the data also challenged existing social model accounts by showing that individual action based on social model principles can lead to attitude change, which can then in turn act as a catalyst for structural change. In other words, it showed that structural change does not always have to be the starting (or end) point in bringing about social change, as most materialist accounts imply. Taking this point together with the previous one, my suggestion is that it is important to promote attitude change simultaneously alongside structural change, in order to move more quickly towards full inclusion. Such an approach is supported by Corker's argument (1999: 636) that structural change alone has not brought about full inclusion for other oppressed groups, and so on its own it is equally unlikely to work for disabled people. Changing the attitudes of non-disabled people also has a role to play, and may on occasion be the catalyst for wider structural change.

Third, the findings suggest that social model writers need to address seriously and systematically the issue of simultaneous oppression (Banton and Hirsch, 2000; Stuart, 1993; Vernon, 1996, 1999). The research uncovered the almost complete absence of people from minority ethnic groups from the setting, from which it could be argued that their experience of exclusion at/from Greenways was even greater than that of white disabled people. This finding disrupted my original expectation that disabled people would be the group facing the most discrimination in the setting, and in turn reinforced my growing conviction that people from a range of minority groups have more in common than we may at first realize, and that forming situational alliances to push for change is a strategy worth pursuing. It also suggested the need to look for ways in which theory in this area may be further developed to support the struggles of activists on the ground.

Fourth, the data shows that people with learning difficulties faced more oppression at Greenways than did those people with physical impairments who were able to join mainstream activity sessions. This highlights the need identified by writers from both social model and learning difficulty fields (Aspis, 1997, 2002; Chappell, 1998; Goodley and Moore, 2000; Chappell, Goodley and Lawthom, 2002; Walmsley, 1997, 2001; Walmsley and Downer, 1997) for more work to be done on making explicit the connections between the experiences of people with learning difficulties and those of other disabled people. All disabled people and our allies have a role to play in this process.

Fifth, while partially supporting calls for an extended social model analysis of impairment, the data also questioned assumptions within both disability and wider sociological theory that everyone is caught up in frantic pursuit of 'the perfect body', and suggested instead that many disabled and non-disabled people look after their bodies to maintain existing basic fitness levels, to minimize further deterioration, or simply because they enjoy sport and leisure activities. As discussed above, I also believe that it is preferable to work towards the inclusion of impairment issues in mainstream sociological analysis of the body, rather than developing a separate sociology of impairment which may simply replicate the assumption of a binary opposition between the experiences of disabled and non-disabled people. Sixth, the data partially supported cultural and psychological explanations for the creation of disabled people as 'other' and as figures of fear or pity to be avoided. This was most marked in the avoidance by some staff and customers of groups of disabled people at the Centre. However, individual disabled people often seemed to be treated in an inclusive way. This suggests that impairment was primarily a factor in 'othering' when combined with presentation as part of a large (and potentially overwhelming) group of disabled people, and the additional complicating factor of the presence of disability professionals who often acted as an intermediary presence between disabled and non-disabled people, thus further reducing the potential for ordinary interactions. Further, if the notion of multiple identities is accepted, in some of which we may be 'insiders' or 'experts', then an analysis which suggests that disabled people are always the 'other' is incorrect. Certainly it does not reflect my own experience of inclusion in the setting, nor that of the other disabled people who visited the site independently.

Overall, in terms of the respective value placed on competing social model accounts, in this study the data support materialist social model explanations that stress the need to remove structural barriers to achieve inclusion. To me, these give the most pragmatic explanations for the creation of disability, and point the way towards eradicating it through the removal of such barriers. At the same time, however, the data also support the general post-structuralist move to deconstruct the notion of an essentialist identity in favour of multiple ones, as a means both of uncovering the multidimensional nature of discrimination against disabled people, and of increasing the potential for disabled people to uncover limited areas of commonality with non-disabled others as a precursor to developing new broader alliances for social change. Perhaps naively, I cannot see what there is to prevent disabled people from drawing on the most useful aspects of both materialist and post-structuralist approaches in their struggles to understand and challenge the socially constructed nature of disability and its effects on their lives, sometimes on our own, and sometimes through alliances with other groups that would help us demonstrate to a wider audience the real disabling nature of social barriers. In turn, I believe this would make more practically achievable Finkelstein's (1996: 11) call for the disabled people's movement to make common cause with other movements for social change as an effective means of challenging the disabling barriers that exclude us all.

Areas where further research is needed

A number of issues have been raised in this study that suggest areas where further research is needed. These include the need to look at ways of further increasing disabled people's participation in sport and leisure activities, and examining the possibilities offered by Frank's concept of the 'communicative body' (1991: 80) in generating meaningful communication between disabled and non-disabled people. The research has also raised some gender and ethical issues, particularly as they relate to disability research. In terms of gender, I have shown that my status as a disabled woman did have an impact on my fieldwork relationships. For the future it would be interesting to compare my experience with that of other disabled women researchers, to see how far matters of gender and sexuality are common issues that are being struggled over. The issue of ethics has also been fundamentally implicated in this research project through my assumption that, as a minority researcher studying members of a majority, I could not simply come straight out and ask non-disabled people what they thought about disabled people, but needed instead to resort to subterfuge and half-truths to elicit their views. For the future, I believe that similar studies are needed across a range of social settings, to confirm, challenge or modify the findings of this research. Additionally, and central to the wider struggle towards inclusive practice, there is a need for more research into how disabled and non-disabled people may be encouraged to start being more honest about their attitudes towards each other, as a precursor to achieving real inclusion. One way in which such research may be facilitated is for disabled and non-disabled researchers to collaborate on inclusion-related projects in the future, and for each to tackle areas of oppressive practice which it may be difficult for the other to address. Thus, as this study has shown, there were elements of my self-presentation in this particular setting which made it possible for me to 'pass' as a person with learning difficulties, and to uncover aspects of their oppression in a way in which I suspect a non-disabled researcher could not have done. On the other hand, there were some fieldwork situations, such as people's avoidance of me through fear, which I could not explore as fully as a non-disabled co-researcher might have been able to. Hence, in working towards inclusion, I believe that there may be great research potential in increased collaboration between disabled and non-disabled researchers, so that a more holistic picture of inclusionary and exclusionary attitudes can be obtained.

General conclusions

When I started this research, I wondered whether social model ideas could be applied more widely. In other words, whether they could be used to show that we are all – differentially – 'disabled people', and that as such we could all use such explanations both to make sense of our individual experiences of oppression, and as a bridge between our experiences and those of others. The data presented here do indeed show that disabled people do not have the monopoly on being oppressed. However, the research has also taught me that ownership of particular labels by specific groups is important. Thus disabled people 'own' disablism. James may be disabled by racism, and women in workforces around Britain are disabled by sexism – but it's the 'dis' we have in common. Words abound to describe minority experience – disempower, disregard, disrespect. In these terms, the word 'disabled' appears far more linguistically negative than the other 'isms', being an explicit descriptor of people rather than simply of power relations. This perhaps reflects a greater negative value judgement by society towards disabled people as a group. In that case, it may be that reclaiming the label for ourselves becomes even more important, rather than seeking to share it with others. And maybe, too, other groups would resist any move to 'diss' their own oppression by seeking to call it something else. Equally, however, I wish to suggest that perhaps in the field of disability studies we need to acknowledge more openly that the social model is only one of a range of explanations for oppression, and to be both less precious about keeping it for ourselves, and more open to making ourselves available to learning from the experience of other movements.

In doing so, we need to be aware that, despite Oliver's statement that the social model was never intended to be a totalizing explanation of disabled people's experience (1996: 31), in reality many of us have been guilty of using it in just this way. It is precisely that tendency which has enabled me to be critical in this book of its supposed omissions and failings, of which I have concentrated a good deal on its implicit assumptions of a binary opposition between disabled and non-disabled people's experiences, and of a straightforward oppressed–oppressor split on impairment grounds. However, just because the social model does not explain the whole of my experience does not mean that I have not found it a powerful tool in helping me to make sense of and resist those situations in which I am oppressed on the grounds of my impairment. Twenty years and more after its original conception, the social model is still extremely relevant to the real lives of disabled people. As such it is a testimony to the vision of those who developed it and who have seen it evolve over time to give an ideas-level response to ever-changing social relationships.

Certainly, I would not wish any of the criticisms made here to detract from that achievement. Still, it was true that in this research, by exposing the different reactions to me generated by my full range of temporal and situational identities, my identity as a disabled person was shown not to be the only important one I had in this setting. Nor was I always a victim of oppression in every situation. Hence it may be argued that some of the assumptions on which the social model is based represent too simplistic an explanation of social relations. The social model does give me an essential explanation of parts of my experience, but not all of it. In part, then, I am arguing here simply for a greater recognition of the limits to the explanatory power of this model, and for the development of more links – both in disability theory and in political practice – between the experience of disabled people and that of people in the wider community, much as black disabled people and gay and lesbian disabled people are already suggesting (Appleby, 1993, 1994; Vernon, 1999).

Indeed, the most important lesson I have taken away from this research is that real inclusion may only be possible once we begin to learn how to engage with each other through dialogues that recognize and value difference. In the world as it is now, a range of groups including women, disabled people, lesbians and gay men, people with little or no money, and people from minority ethnic groups face daily structural and attitude discrimination in their lives, because of who they are in relation to others who have more power than them. Writing from a broad social justice perspective, both Phillips (1999) and Taylor (1992) have emphasized the huge dangers involved in perpetuating the traditional mainstream approach of failing to recognize that people are different from each other, and of instead seeing only the person with less cultural and economic power as being different from the more powerful other. They argue that such an exclusionary approach merely reinforces existing inequalities, and may lead to the attempted assimilation of the individual or minority group into the cultural and political norms imposed by the majority. Instead, both writers see the way forward towards real social inclusion as depending on our ability to learn to engage in dialogues that acknowledge and respect people's differences from each other, and which do not require the ultimate capitulation of one party to the other in the way that traditional hierarchical approaches have done. Their suggestions are particularly relevant now, as social movements continue to grow (Giddens, 1991; Giroux, 1992). In this climate it is unlikely that members of minority groups will continue to tolerate their difference being viewed in a negative way by the mainstream. So, what can policy makers, practitioners and theorists do to keep pace with such developments?

Taking my lead from Phillips (1999) and Taylor (1992), I believe that true inclusion will only be achieved when as a society we begin to systematically build all social provision around the premise of the equal valuing of difference. In this respect, it may be helpful for disability theorists and practitioners to compare their approaches to inclusion with those of writers concerned with issues of social justice as they relate to members of other minority groups in Western societies, and to see what lessons can be drawn from such comparisons. We may then be in a stronger position to push for disabled people's experience of exclusion to be tackled in the same systemic way as that proposed for those other minorities. Applying a 'valuing difference' approach to the way that society views disabled people thus necessitates that we challenge the assumption that impairment automatically results in devalued social status. Instead, we need to follow the lead of the disabled people's movement in encouraging more disabled people to acknowledge and celebrate their own difference from the norm. By such means may we begin to move towards achieving inclusion on our own terms.

References

Abberley, P. (1987) 'The concept of oppression and the development of a social theory of disability', *Disability, Handicap and Society*, 2: 5–19.

Abberley, P. (1997) 'The limits of classical social theory in the analysis and transformation of disablement – (can this really be the end, to be stuck inside of Mobile with the Memphis Blues again?)', in L. Barton and M. Oliver (eds) *Disability Studies: Past, Present and Future*, Leeds: Disability Press, 25–44.

Anon (1998) 'Hi-de-bye Bye', *Disability Now*, November issue.

Appleby, Y. (1993) 'Disability and compulsory heterosexuality', in S. Wilkinson and C. Kitzinger (eds) *Heterosexuality: A Feminism and Psychology Reader*, London: Sage, 266–9.

Appleby, Y. (1994) 'Out in the margins', *Disability and Society*, 9: 19–32.

Aspis, S. (1997) 'Self-advocacy for people with learning difficulties: does it have a future?', *Disability and Society*, 12: 647–54.

Aspis, S. (1999) 'What they don't tell disabled people with learning difficulties', in M. Corker and S. French (eds) *Disability Discourse*, Buckingham: Open University Press, 173–82.

Aspis, S. (2002) 'Self-advocacy: vested interests and misunderstandings', *British Journal of Learning Disabilities*, 30: 3–7.

Bagihole, B. (1997) *Equal Opportunities and Social Policy: Issues of Gender, Race and Disability*, London: Longman.

Banton, M., and Hirsch, M. (2000) *Double Invisibility: A Study into the Needs of Black Disabled People in Warwickshire*, Coventry: Council of Disabled People.

Barnes, C. (1991) *Disabled People in Britain and Discrimination: A Case for Anti-discrimination Legislation*, London: Hurst and Co.

Barnes, C. (1996) 'Theories of disability and the origins of the oppression of disabled people in western society', in L. Barton (ed.) *Disability and Society: Emerging Issues and Insights*, London: Longman, 43–60.

Barnes, C., Mercer, G., and Shakespeare, T. (1999) *Exploring Disability: A Sociological Introduction*, Cambridge: Polity Press.

Barton, L. (1993) 'The struggle for citizenship: the case of disabled people', *Disability and Society*, 8: 236–48.

Borthwick, C. (1996) 'Racism, IQ and Down syndrome', *Disability and Society*, 11: 403–10.

Brown, H. (1992) 'Working with staff around sexuality and power', in A. Waitman and S. Conboy-Hill (eds) *Psychotherapy and Mental Handicap*, London: Sage, 185–201.

Brown, H., and Smith, H. (eds) (1992) *Normalisation: A Reader for the 1990s*, London: Routledge.

BT/The Fieldfare Trust (1997) *BT Countryside for All Standards and Guidelines: A Good Practice Guide to Disabled People's Access to the Countryside*, Barnsley: Ledgard and Jepson.

Campbell, J., and Oliver, M. (1996) *Disability Politics: Understanding our Past, Changing our Future*, London: Routledge.

Carr, W., and Kemmis, S. (1986) *Becoming Critical: Education, Knowledge and Action Research*, London: Falmer Press.

Casling, D. (1993) 'Cobblers and song-birds: the language and imagery of disability', *Disability, Handicap and Society*, 8: 203–10.

Chappell, A.L. (1998) 'Still out in the cold: people with learning difficulties and the social model of disability', in T. Shakespeare (ed.) *The Disability Reader: Social Science Perspectives*, London: Cassell, 211–20.

Chappell, A.L., Goodley, D., and Lawthom, R. (2002) 'Making connections: the relevance of the social model of disability for people with learning difficulties', *British Journal of Learning Disabilities*, 29: 45–50.

Charles, H. (1992) 'Whiteness – the relevance of politically colouring the "non"', in H. Hinds, A. Phoenix and J. Stacey (eds) *Working Out: New Directions for Women's Studies*, London: Falmer Press, 29–35.

Clough, P. (1996) '"Again fathers and sons": the mutual construction of self, story and special educational needs', *Disability and Society*, 11: 71–81.

Clough, P., and Barton, L. (eds) (1998) *Articulating with Difficulty: Research Voices in Inclusive Education*, London: Paul Chapman Publishing.

Coffey A (1999) *The Ethnographic Self: Fieldwork and the Representation of Identity*, London: Sage.

Cohen, L., and Manion, L. (1994) *Research Methods in Education*, London: Routledge.

Conboy-Hill, S. (1992) 'Grief, loss and people with learning disabilities', in A. Waitman and S. Conboy-Hill (eds) *Psychotherapy and Mental Handicap*, London: Sage, 150–70.

Connolly, P. (1996) 'Doing what comes naturally? Standpoint epistemology, critical social research and the politics of identity', in E.S. Ingram and J. Busfield (eds) *Methodological Imaginations*, Basingstoke: Macmillan, 185–99.

Corbett, J. (1994) 'A proud label: exploring the relationship between disability politics and gay pride', *Disability and Society*, 9: 343–57.

Corker, M. (1999) 'Differences, conflations and foundations: the limits to "accurate" theoretical representation of disabled people's experience?', *Disability and Society*, 14: 627–42.

Crow, L. (1996) 'Including all of our lives: renewing the social model of disability', in J. Morris (ed.) *Encounters with Strangers: Feminism and Disability*, London: Women's Press, 206–26.

Dalley, G. (1992) 'Social welfare ideologies and normalization: links and conflicts', in H. Brown and H. Smith (eds) *Normalization: A Reader for the 1990s*, London: Routledge, 100–11.

Department for Education and Skills (1999) *A Fresh Start*, London: HMSO.

Department of Health (1989) *Caring for People – Community Care in the Next Decade and Beyond*, Command 849, London: HMSO.

Department of Health (2001) *Valuing People – A New Strategy for Learning Disability for the 21st Century*, London: HMSO.

Department of Health and Social Security (1971) *Better Services for the Mentally Handicapped*, Command 4683, London: HMSO.

Department of Health and Social Security (1981) *Care in the Community – A Consultative Document on Moving Resources for Care in England*, London: HMSO.

Disability Discrimination Act (1995) London: HMSO.

Disabled People's (Employment) Act (1944) London: HMSO.

Douard, J.W. (1995) 'Disability and the persistence of the "normal"', in S. Kay and D. Barnard (eds) *Chronic Illness: From Experience to Policy*, Indiana: Indiana University Press.

Dowse, L. (2001) 'Contesting practices, challenging codes: self-advocacy, disability politics and the social model', *Disability and Society*, 16: 123–41.

Eagly, A.H., and Chaiken, S. (1993) *The Psychology of Attitudes*, London: Harcourt Brace College Publishers.

Education (Handicapped Children) Act 1970, London: HMSO.

Erevelles, N. (1996) 'Disability and the dialectics of difference', *Disability and Society*, 11: 519–37.

Finch, J. (1993) 'It's great to have someone to talk to: ethics and politics of interviewing women', in M. Hammersley (ed.) *Social Research: Philosophy, Politics and Practice*, London: Sage, 166–80.

Fine, M. (1994) 'Working the hyphens: reinventing self and other in qualitative research', in N.K. Denzin and Y.S. Lincoln (eds) *Handbook of Qualitative Research*, London: Sage, 70–82.

Finger, A. (1991) *Past Due: A Story of Disability, Pregnancy and Birth*, London: Women's Press.

Finkelstein, V. (1980) *Attitudes and Disabled People: Issues for Discussion*, New York: World Rehabilitation Fund.

Finkelstein, V. (1996) 'The disability movement has run out of steam', *Disability Now*, February, p. 11.

Fishbein, M., and Azjen, I. (1975) *Belief, Attitude, Intention and Behavior: An Introduction to Theory and Research*, London: Addison-Wesley Publishing Company.

Frank, A. (1991) 'For a sociology of the body', in M. Featherstone, M. Hepworth, and B.S. Turner (eds) *The Body: Social Processes and Cultural Theory*, London: Sage, 36–101.

Gabel, S. (1999) 'Depressed and disabled: some discursive problems with mental illness', in M. Corker and S. French, *Disability Discourse*, Buckingham: Open University Press, 38–46.

Gelb, S.A. (1987) 'Social deviance and the "discovery" of the moron', *Disability, Handicap and Society*, 2: 247–58.

Germon, P. (1999) '"Purely academic"? Exploring the relationship between theory and political activism', *Disability and Society*, 14: 687–92.

Giddens, A. (1991) *Modernity and Self-identity: Self and Society in the Late Modern Age*, Oxford: Polity Press.

Gillborn, D. (1990) *'Race', Ethnicity and Education: Teaching and Learning in Multi-ethnic Schools*, London: Unwin Hyman.

Gillborn, D., and Youdell, D. (2000) *Rationing Education: Policy, Practice, Reform and Equity*, Buckingham: Open University Press.

Gilman, S. (1997) 'The deep structure of stereotypes', in S. Hall (ed.) *Representation: Cultural Representations and Signifying Practices*, Milton Keynes: Open University Press, 284–5.

Giroux, H. (1992) *Border Crossings: Cultural Workers and the Politics of Education*, London: Routledge.

Glassner, B. (1992) *Bodies: Overcoming the Tyranny of Perfection*, Los Angeles: Lowell House.

Goffman, E. (1990) *Stigma: Notes on the Management of Spoiled Identity*, Harmondsworth; Penguin.

Goodley, D., and Moore, M. (2000) 'Doing disability research: activist lives and the academy', *Disability and Society*, 15: 861–82.

Greater Manchester Coalition of Disabled People (1999) GMCDP *Information Bulletin*, July, p. 1.

Greater Manchester Coalition of Disabled People (2000) GMCDP *Where Have All the Activists Gone? Special Issue*.

Griffin, C., and Wetherell, M. (eds) (1992) 'Feminist psychology and the study of men: part II: politics and practice', *Feminism and Psychology: An International Journal*, 133–68.

Hall, S. (1997) 'The spectacle of the Other', in S. Hall (ed.) *Representation: Cultural Representations and Signifying Practices*, Milton Keynes: Open University Press, 223–90.

Hammersley, M. (1998) *Reading Ethnographic Research: A Critical Guide*, London: Longman.

Hammersley, M., and Atkinson, P. (1983) *Ethnography: Principles in Practice*, London: Tavistock Publications.

Henwood, K.L. and Pidgeon, N.F. (1993) 'Qualitative research and psychological theorizing', in M. Hammersley (ed.) *Social Research: Philosophy, Politics and Practice*, London: Sage, 14–32.

Hevey, D. (ed.) (1992) *The Creatures Time Forgot: Photography and Disability Imagery*, London: Routledge.

Hockenberry, J. (1996) *Declarations of Independence: War Zones and Wheelchairs*, London: Viking.

Home Office (1999) *The Stephen Lawrence Inquiry: Report of an Inquiry by Sir William MacPherson of Cluny*, Command 4262–I, London: HMSO.

hooks, bell (2000) *Feminist Theory: From Margin to Center*, London: Pluto Press.

Hughes, B. (2000) 'Medicine and aesthetic invalidation of disabled people', *Disability and Society*, 15: 555–68.

Hughes, B., and Paterson, K. (1997) 'The social model of disability and the disappearing body: towards a sociology of impairment', *Disability and Society*, 12: 325–40.

Humphrey, J.C. (2000) 'Researching disability politics, or, some problems with the social model in practice', *Disability and Society*, 15: 63–85.

Johnston, M. (1996) 'Models of disability', *Psychologist*, 9: 205–10.

King's Fund (1980) *An Ordinary Life – Comprehensive Locally Based Services for Mentally Handicapped People*, London: King's Fund Centre.

King's Fund (1984) *An Ordinary Working Life – Vocational Services for People with Mental Handicaps*, King's Fund Project Paper No 50, London: King's Fund Centre.

Kitzinger, C., and Wilkinson, S. (1993) 'Theorizing heterosexuality', in S. Wilkinson and C. Kitzinger (eds) *Heterosexuality: A Feminism and Psychology Reader*, London: Sage, 1–32.

Kitzinger, C., and Wilkinson, S. (1994) 'Virgins and queers: rehabilitating heterosexuality', *Gender and Society*, 8: 444–62.

MacFarlane, A. (1994) 'Subtle forms of abuse and their long term effects', *Disability and Society*, 9: 85–88.

Manion, M.L., and Bersani, H.A. (1987) 'Mental retardation as a Western sociological construct: a cross-cultural analysis', *Disability, Handicap and Society*, 2: 231–45.

Marks, D. (1999a) *Disability: Controversial Debates and Psychosocial Perspectives*, London: Routledge.

Marks, D. (1999b) 'Dimensions of oppression: theorising the embodied subject', *Disability and Society*, 14: 611–26.

Mason, M., and Rieser, R. (1999) *Altogether Better (from 'Special Needs' to Equality in Education)*, London: Charity Projects/Comic Relief.

Mohanty, C.T. (1995) 'Feminist encounters: locating the politics of experience', in L. Nicholson and S. Seidman (eds) *Social Postmodernism: Beyond Identity Politics*, New York: Cambridge University Press, 68–86.

Morris, J. (1991) *Pride Against Prejudice*, London: Women's Press.

Morris, J. (1993) *Independent Lives? Community Care and Disabled People*, Basingstoke: Macmillan.

Morris, J. (ed.) (1996) *Encounters With Strangers: Feminism and Disability*, London: Women's Press.

Mouffe, C. (1995) 'Feminism, citizenship and radical democratic politics', in L. Nicholson and S. Seidman (eds) *Social Postmodernism: Beyond Identity Politics*, New York: Cambridge University Press, 315–31.

Murray, P. (2002) *Hello! Are You Listening? – Disabled Teenagers' Experience of Access to Leisure*, York: Joseph Rowntree Foundation.

Obholzer, A., and Zagier Roberts, V. (1994) *The Unconscious at Work: Individual and Organizational Stress in the Human Services*, London: Routledge.

Oliver, M. (1990) *The Politics of Disablement*, Basingstoke: Macmillan.

Oliver, M. (1996) *Understanding Disability: From Theory to Practice*, Basingstoke: Macmillan.

Oliver, M. (1997) 'Emancipatory research: realistic goal or impossible dream?', in C. Barnes and G. Mercer (eds) *Doing Disability Research*, Leeds: Disability Press, 15–32 .

Ozga, J., and Gewirtz, S. (1994) 'Sex, lies and audiotape: interviewing the education policy elite', in D. Halpin and B. Troyna (eds) *Researching Education Policy: Ethical and Methodological Issues*, London: Falmer Press, 121–36.

Paterson, K., and Hughes, B. (1999) 'Disability studies and phenomenology: the carnal politics of everyday life', *Disability and Society*, 14: 597–610.

Phelan, S. (1995) 'The space of justice: lesbians and democratic politics', in L. Nicholson and S. Seidman (eds) *Social Postmodernism: Beyond Identity Politics*, New York: Cambridge University Press, 332–56.

Phillips, A. (1999) *Which Equalities Matter?* Oxford: Blackwell.

Priestley, M. (1995) 'Commonality and difference in the movement: an "Association of Blind Asians" in Leeds', *Disability and Society*, 10: 157–69.

Priestley, M. (1998) 'Constructions and creations: idealism, materialism and disability theory', *Disability and Society*, 13: 75–94.

Race D.G. (1999) *Social Role Valorization and the English Experience*, Wilding and Birch: London.

Rattansi, A. (1995) 'Just framing: ethnicities and racism in a "post-modern" framework', in L. Nicholson and S. Seidman (eds) *Social Postmodernism: Beyond Identity Politics* New York: Cambridge University Press, 250–86.

Schein, E.H. (1987) *The Clinical Perspective in Fieldwork*, London: Sage.

Scull, A. (1993) *The Most Solitary of Afflictions: Madness and Society in Britain 1700–1900*, London: Yale University Press.

Seidman, S. (1995) 'Deconstructing queer theory or the undertheorization of the social and the ethical', in L. Nicholson and S. Seidman (eds) *Social Postmodernism: Beyond Identity Politics*, New York: Cambridge University Press, 116–41.

Shakespeare, T. (1994) 'Cultural representation of disabled people: dustbins for disavowal?', *Disability and Society*, 9: 283–301.

Shilling, C. (1993) *The Body and Social Theory*, London: Sage.

Silverman, D. (1993) *Interpreting Qualitative Data: Methods for Analysing Talk, Text and Interaction*, London: Sage.

Simons, K. (1992) *Sticking up for Yourself: Self-advocacy and People with Learning Difficulties*, York: Joseph Rowntree Foundation.

Sinason, V. (1992) *Mental Handicap and the Human Condition: New Approaches from the Tavistock*, London: Free Association Books.

Smith, H., and Brown, H. (1992) 'Inside-out: a psychodynamic approach to normalisation', in H. Brown and H. Smith (eds) *Normalisation: A Reader for the 1990s*, London: Routledge, 84–99.

Somers, M. (1994) 'The narrative constitution of identity: a relational and network approach', *Theory and Society*, 23: 605–49.

Sparkes, A.C. (1994) 'Life histories and the issue of voice: reflections on an emerging relationship', *Qualitative Studies in Education*, 7: 165–83.

Sparkes, A.C. (1995) 'Writing people: reflections on the dual crises of representation and legitimation in qualitative inquiry', *QUEST*, 47: 158–95.

Sparkes, A.C. (1996) 'The fatal flaw: a narrative of the fragile body-self', *Qualitative Inquiry*, 2: 463–94.

St Claire, L. (1986) 'Mental retardation: impairment or handicap?', *Disability, Handicap and Society*, 1: 233–43.

Stanley, L., and Wise, S. (1993) *Breaking Out Again: Feminist Ontology and Epistemology*, London: Routledge.

Stone, S.D. (1995) 'The myth of bodily perfection', *Disability and Society*, 10: 413–24.

Stuart, O. (1993) 'Double oppression: an appropriate starting point?', in J. Swain, V. Finkelstein, S. French and M. Oliver (eds) *Disabling Barriers, Enabling Environments*, Buckingham: Open University Press, 93–100.

Sutherland, A. (1981) *Disabled We Stand*, London: Souvenir Press.

Swain, J. (1993) 'Taught helplessness? Or a say for disabled students in schools', in J. Swain, V. Finkelstein, S. French and M. Oliver (eds) *Disabling Barriers, Enabling Environments*, Buckingham: Open University Press, 155–62.

Swain, J., and French, S. (2000) 'Towards an affirmatory model of disability', *Disability and Society*, 15: 569–82.

Symington, N. (1992) 'Countertransference with mentally handicapped clients', in A. Waitman and S. Conboy-Hill (eds) *Psychotherapy and Mental Handicap*, London: Sage, 132–38.

Szivos, S. (1992) 'The limits to integration?', in H. Brown and H. Smith (eds) *Normalisation: A Reader for the 1990s*, London: Routledge, 112–33.

Tarver-Behring, S. (1994) 'White women's identity and diversity: awareness from the inside-out', in K. Bhavanani and A. Phoenix (eds) *Shifting Identities, Shifting Racisms: A Feminism and Psychology Reader*, London: Sage, 206–8.

Taylor, C. (1992) *Multiculturalism and 'The Politics of Recognition'*, Princeton: Princeton University Press.

Thomas, C. (1999) *Female Forms: Experiencing and Understanding Disability*, Buckingham: Open University Press.

Torkildsen, G. (1993) *Torkildsen's Guides to Leisure Management*, Harlow: Longman.

Tregaskis, C. (1998) 'Life beyond paid employment: disabled women's experiences of giving up work', unpublished dissertation in partial fulfilment of MA in Disability Studies, University of Sheffield.

Trepagnier, B. (1994) 'The politics of white and black bodies', in K. Bhavanani and A. Phoenix (eds) *Shifting Identities, Shifting Racisms: A Feminism and Psychology Reader*, London: Sage, 199–205.

Turner, B.S. (1992) *Regulating Bodies: Essays in Medical Sociology*, London: Routledge.

Tyne, A. (1992) 'Normalisation: from theory to practice', in H. Brown and H. Smith (eds) *Normalisation: A Reader for the 1990s*, London: Routledge, 35–46.

UPIAS (1976) *Fundamental Principles of Disability*, London: Union of the Physically Impaired Against Segregation.

Vernon, A. (1996) 'Fighting two different battles: unity is preferable to enmity', *Disability and Society*, 11: 285–90.

Vernon, A. (1999) 'The dialectics of multiple identities and the disabled people's movement', *Disability and Society*, 14: 385–98.

Walmsley, J. (1997) 'Including people with learning difficulties: theory and practice', in L. Barton and M. Oliver (eds) *Disability Studies: Past, Present and Future*, Leeds: Disability Press, 62–77.

Walmsley, J. (2001) 'Normalization, emancipatory research and inclusive research in learning disability', *Disability and Society*, 16: 187–205.

Walmsley, J., and Downer, J. (1997) 'Shouting the loudest: self-advocacy, power and diversity', in P. Ramcharan, G. Roberts, G. Grant and J. Borland (eds) *Empowerment in Everyday Life: Learning Difficulty*, London: Jessica Kingsley, 35–47.

Warren, N., and Jahoda, M. (eds) (1976) *Attitudes: Selected Readings*, Harmondsworth: Penguin.

Whitehead, S. (1992) 'The social origins of normalization', in H. Brown and H. Smith (eds) *Normalisation: A Reader for the 1990s*, London: Routledge, 47–59.

Wilkinson, S., and Kitzinger, C. (1996) *Representing the Other: A Feminism and Psychology Reader*, London: Sage.

Williams, L., and Nind, M. (1999) 'Insiders or outsiders: normalisation and women with learning difficulties', 14: 659–72.

Wolfensberger, W. (1992) *A Brief Introduction to Social Role Valorization as a High-order Concept for Structuring Human Services*, Syracuse, NY: Training Institute for Human Service Planning, Leadership and Change Agency (Syracuse University).

Wolfensberger, W. and Tullman, S. (1989) 'A brief outline of the principle of normalization', in A. Brechin and J. Walmsley (eds) *Making Connections: Reflecting on the Lives and Experiences of People with Learning Difficulties*, Sevenoaks: Hodder & Stoughton.

Wong, L.M. (1994) 'Di(s)-secting and dis(s)-closing "whiteness": two tales about psychology', in K. Bhavanani and A. Phoenix (eds) *Shifting Identities, Shifting Racisms: A Feminism and Psychology Reader*, London: Sage, 133–53.

Young, I.M. (1995) 'Gender as seriality: thinking about women as a social collective', in L. Nicholson and S. Seidman (eds) *Social Postmodernism: Beyond Identity Politics*, New York: Cambridge University Press, 187–215.

Zarb, G. (1992) 'On the road to Damascus: first steps towards changing the relations of research production', *Disability, Handicap and Society*, 7: 125–38.

Zarb, G. (1997) 'Researching disabling barriers', in C. Barnes and G. Mercer (eds) *Doing Disability Research*, Leeds: Disability Press.

Index

305.9   Tregaskis, Claire,
Tre   1962-

          Constructions of
          disability.

DATE			